CIRCULATORY PHYSIOLOGY

—the essentials

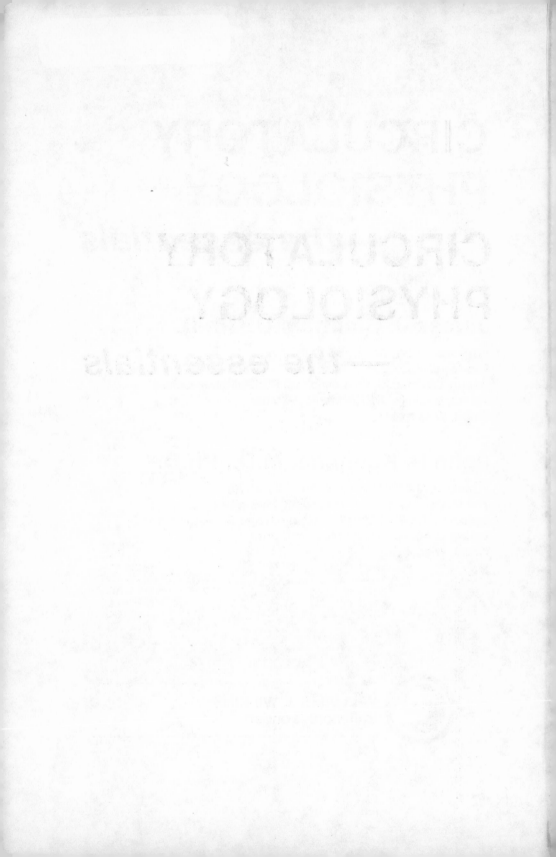

CIRCULATORY PHYSIOLOGY
—the essentials

James J. Smith, M.D., Ph.D.
Professor of Physiology and Medicine
The Medical College of Wisconsin, Milwaukee
Deputy Director, Cardiopulmonary Rehabilitation Center
Veterans Administration Medical Center
Wood, Wisconsin

John P. Kampine, M.D., Ph.D.
Professor of Anesthesiology and Physiology
The Medical College of Wisconsin, Milwaukee
Associate Chief of Staff for Research and Development
Veterans Administration Medical Center
Wood, Wisconsin

WILLIAMS & WILKINS
Baltimore/London

Library of Congress Cataloging in Publication Data

Smith, James John, 1914-
    Circulatory physiology—the essentials.

    Includes index.
    1. Cardiovascular system. 2. Blood—Circulation. 3. Cardiovascular system—Dis-
eases. I. Kampine, John P., joint author. II. Title. [DNLM: 1. Blood circulation.
WG103 S651c]
QP102.S64   612′.1   79-11076
ISBN 0-683-07885-2

Composed and printed at the
Waverly Press, Inc.
Mt. Royal and Guilford Aves.
Baltimore, Md. 21202, U.S.A.

Dedicated to our parents

James W. and   and   Dr. Clifford and
Catherine Smith   Florence Kampine

They showed us the way.

Preface

This book—which is intended for medical students—has evolved from our lectures in cardiovascular physiology to the medical and graduate classes. However, we have also been influenced in the method of presentation by our teaching sessions with nurses and allied health students as well as with residents and physician groups. It seems that all of us share the perennial problem of the increasing volume of material and the pressing need to cull out the relevant in the time allotted. As a consequence we have tried to confine ourselves to the essentials.

We had two primary aims in the preparation of this book; the first was to present the basics of circulatory physiology mainly for those who are (or will be) charged with the diagnosis and care of cardiovascular patients. As a result, many interesting topics dealing with fundamental mechanisms have usually been omitted or treated only briefly. In further accord with this objective, clinical applications have been emphasized throughout the text and two chapters on the pathophysiology of certain cardiovascular disorders have been included. Physicians and others involved with coronary care units and circulatory stress testing may find this approach useful.

A second objective has been to develop some of the more difficult concepts in an orderly, stepwise and hopefully intelligible manner. Diagrams have been liberally used and physical, chemical and biological principles and analogies incorporated when they seemed useful.

In developing topics rather briefly and bypassing some of the complex issues, the danger is that the student may feel that the subject is straightforward and that most problems are resolved, which of course is far from the truth. Not only on questions of diagnosis and treatment but on a number of basic concepts, there is still intensive investigation and considerable controversy.

But it is sometimes helpful to have a small-scale map of the battle-field, which is why we undertook to write this book. And, in any event, for the student, the classroom and the laboratory may be better places to air the unsolved problems. We also hope that the references we have included, many of them reviews by leading authorities, will help to focus attention on current research in this field.

We wish to acknowledge, with very real gratitude, our many colleagues and our own students who have made helpful comments and valuable suggestions. However, in the final analysis, the selection of content and method of presentation must be our own responsibility; such selection is a highly individual process and no doubt others would have made different choices. We would, therefore, very much welcome comments, not only regarding specific errors or omissions but also general impressions and suggestions.

James J. Smith   *John P. Kampine*

Acknowledgments

In a field as broad as circulatory physiology, it has become difficult to prepare a textbook without considerable help. We received not only help but encouragement from many people and to them goes our sincerest gratitude. A number of faculty from different disciplines were kind enough to check parts of the manuscript and make suggestions. From the faculty of other universities we gratefully acknowledge the help of Dr. James P. Filkins and Dr. Walter C. Randall of the Stritch School of Medicine, Dr. Francis J. Haddy of the Uniformed Services University, Dr. Dean C. Jeutter of Marquette University, Dr. Richard A. Kenney of George Washington University, Dr. John B. West of the University of California, San Diego, Dr. Kenneth E. Penrod of the University of Florida, Dr. Robert W. Rasch of East Tennessee State University, Dr. Keith E. Cooper of the University of Calgary, and Dr. John Naughton, State University of New York, Buffalo.

Members of our own faculty at The Medical College of Wisconsin contributed greatly with advice on specific chapters and portions of the manuscript. Among these were Dr. David G. Kamper, Dr. Lois M. Sheldahl, Dr. Mohendr S. Kochar, Dr. Michael E. Korns, Dr. Michael J. Hosko, Jr., Dr. Donald P. Schleuter, Dr. V. R. Bamrah, Dr. C. Vincent Hughes, Dr. Michael H. Keelan, Jr., Dr. Christopher A. Dawson, Dr. Donal Pedersen, Dr. William J. Gallen, Dr. Felix E. Tristani, Dr. Harold L. Brooks, Dr. H. David Friedberg, Dr. Peter Hanson, Dr. James Leibsohn and Dr. Basil T. Doumas.

We want to extend our very special thanks to several physiologists who critically reviewed substantial portions of the manuscript and made very valuable suggestions; these were Dr. William V. Judy of the University of Indiana School of Medicine, Dr. Joseph R. Logic of the University of Alabama Medical Center, Dr. Peter A. Kot of Georgetown University School of Medicine, Dr. V. Thomas Wiedmeier, Medical College of Georgia and from our own faculty, Dr. William J. Stekiel, Dr. David F. Stowe and Dr. Jeanne L. Seagard. To these "special consultants" we are most grateful; their comments were exceedingly helpful.

We are most happy to acknowledge the outstanding skill of Carole Hilmer, our medical artist who prepared the diagrams, the excellent typing assistance of Helen Russell and the assistance of Mr. George E. Spuda, Chief Medical Media Service, Veterans Administration Medical Center, Wood, Wisconsin. Our thanks also to Thomas J. Ebert who planned some of the diagrams and Lucille Maney for a big assist in preparing copy.

We have—with intent—reserved until last our tribute to two people who, without question, gave service well "beyond the call" in the production of this book. Carole Graff, skillfully and tirelessly oversaw the typing and assembly of the entire manuscript; with patience and foresight she steered us through. And also to her colleague, Jill Reinke, our deepest appreciation; versatile and indispensable, Jill helped with planning of the diagrams and coordination of the entire effort.

While we take pleasure in acknowledging the assistance of our colleagues, we of course, take full responsibility for any errors or omissions in the manuscript.

CONTENTS

CHAPTER 3. THE HEART: STRUCTURE AND FUNCTION

CHAPTER 4. PRESSURE AND FLOW IN THE ARTERIAL AND VENOUS SYSTEMS

CHAPTER 5. ELECTRICAL PROPERTIES OF THE HEART

CHAPTER 6. CONTRACTILE PROPERTIES OF THE HEART

CHAPTER 7. VENOUS RETURN AND CARDIAC OUTPUT

CHAPTER 8. THE MICROCIRCULATION AND THE LYMPHATIC SYSTEM

CHAPTER 9. THE PERIPHERAL CIRCULATION AND ITS REGULATION

CHAPTER 10. REGULATION OF ARTERIAL BLOOD PRESSURE

CHAPTER 11. CIRCULATION TO SPECIAL REGIONS

CHAPTER 12. PHYSIOLOGY OF EXERCISE AND THE EFFECT OF AGING

CHAPTER 13. CIRCULATORY RESPONSE TO NON-EXERCISE STRESS

CHAPTER 14. PATHOPHYSIOLOGY: ISCHEMIC HEART DISEASE AND CONGESTIVE HEART FAILURE

CHAPTER 15. PATHOPHYSIOLOGY: HYPERTENSION AND CIRCULATORY SHOCK

chapter 1

Blood and the Circulation: General Features

GENERAL CHARACTERISTICS

In man, as well as in higher animals, the circulation plays a special role. It is the transport system for the delivery of oxygen and the removal of carbon dioxide and this carrier function makes it indispensable for the survival of every cell and organ of the body. The circulation also delivers nutrients from the gastrointestinal tract to all the body parts, carries waste products of cellular metabolism to the kidney and other excretory organs, transports electrolytes and important chemical regulators called hormones, and serves to maintain body temperature. In addition, it is instrumental in converting certain inactive materials into active compounds and transports cells and immune substances which are concerned with the defense mechanisms of the body.

Since the storage capacity of tissues for oxygen is small, the body requires an adequate minute by minute supply. Under ordinary circumstances the survival times of the "vital organs," *i.e.,* the brain and heart, without oxygen, are only a few minutes, so that even a brief

1

failure of the circulatory or respiratory system may have a serious or fatal outcome.

Another significant characteristic of the circulatory system is its vulnerability to disease. The incidence of cardiovascular disorders is particularly high in the so-called "developed" nations of the western world. While rheumatic and coronary heart disease as well as cerebro-vascular accidents (stroke) have become prevalent, the most common of all circulatory disorders is hypertension—with over 33 million cases at present in the United States.

Of the current annual two million deaths in the United States, 52% are the result of cardiovascular disease—more than cancer (15%), trauma (6%) and all other causes combined. The majority of these deaths are associated with atherosclerosis of the coronary, cerebral or renal arteries; although the specific cause of atherosclerotic disease is unknown, major "risk factors" such as high blood pressure, cigarette smoking and increased blood cholesterol are known to predispose. A world-wide research and educational effort has been mounted in recent years in an attempt to deal with the immense problem of cardiovas-cular disease.

FUNCTIONAL DIVISIONS OF THE CIRCULATION

There are two main components of the circulation, the smaller pulmonary division consisting of the pulmonary artery, capillaries and pulmonary veins, and the much larger systemic division, consisting of the aorta, arterial branches, capillaries, veins and vena cavae; the systemic vessels supply and drain all the organs and tissues of the body. These two divisions are serially-connected hydraulic circuits and form a closed system; each consists of a pump, a distributing system, an exchange system and a collecting system (Fig. 1–1). Whereas the two divisions function in a generally similar manner they have some important differences; the pulmonary division has a much lesser vol-ume, its vessels are shorter and thinner walled and it operates under lower pressure and with less resistance to flow.

The *heart* provides the propulsive force for both divisions and has four chambers—a right and left atrium and a right and left ventricle (Fig. 1–2). The atria are, in essence, auxiliary pumps which assist the flow of blood into the ventricles and help fill these chambers properly so they will be better primed for the subsequent power stroke. The

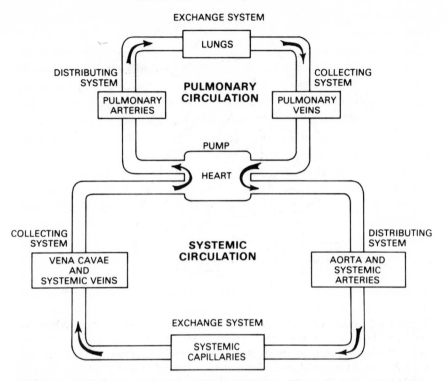

Figure 1-1. Functional divisions of the circulation. The pulmonary circulation delivers blood to the lungs for the elimination of carbon dioxide and the acquisition of oxygen. The systemic circulation transports oxygen (as well as nutrients and other substances) to all the tissues of the body.

ventricles are the main pump elements; the right ventricle propels blood through the pulmonary artery to the lungs (pulmonary circulation) and the left ventricle through the aorta and systemic arteries to the remainder of the body (systemic circulation). Each ventricular chamber has inlet and outlet valves which act reciprocally, that is, one closes before the other opens, thus preventing backflow.

The left ventricle is a high pressure pump; during contraction of its muscular wall (called systole), a peak internal pressure of about 120 mm Hg is produced, which falls to near zero pressure during the subsequent resting or filling phase (diastole). As a consequence the systolic and diastolic pressures of the left ventricle are designated as

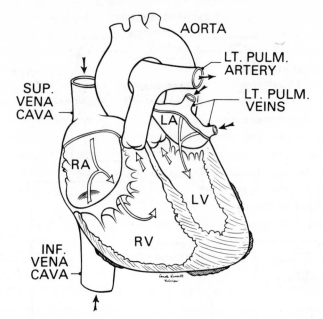

Figure 1-2. Right and left side of the heart (semi-diagrammatic). When the right and left atria contract, they propel blood into the respective ventricles. When the latter contract, the right ventricle forces blood toward the lungs and the left toward the periphery. All the valves—the right and left atrioventricular (AV) valves and the pulmonary and aortic valves—are unidirectional. With the onset of systole both ventricles contract simultaneously, the AV valves close, the aortic and pulmonary valves open and blood is ejected. Note the greater wall thickness of the left ventricle.

120/0. The right ventricle is a low pressure pump and its corresponding pressures during systole and diastole are about 25/0. Normally, the two ventricles are in almost identical phase and rhythm because they are compressed simultaneously by the muscular myocardium which envelops both chambers. The myocardium of the left ventricle is usually 8 to 10 mm thick, that of the right ventricle about 2 to 3 mm. Since the overlying muscle mass is an important factor in determining the internal pressure developed in a hollow organ, it is logical that the ratio of the peak internal pressures of the two ventricles would be similar to the ratio of their muscle thicknesses.

Distributing System. The arteries are branched, hollow cylindrical tubes. In the systemic division, the aorta (the largest artery) and its arterial branches are long, rather thick-walled, high pressure conduits which transport blood over the systemic circuit to the small arteries and arterioles. Their internal pressure diminishes from about 120 mm Hg (systolic) and 80 mm Hg (diastolic) at the beginning of the aorta to a constant mean pressure of about 25 mm Hg at the arteriolar end of the capillaries. The pulmonary artery pressure, normally about 25/10 mm Hg, decreases to a mean pressure of about 10 mm Hg at the entrance to the lung capillaries. Aside from blood distribution, the arterial systems have two additional, important functions; the first portions serve a pressure-storing or "windkessel" function and the terminal arteries, a resistance or "stopcock" function. These are described later in this chapter.

Exchange System. Capillaries are numerous, tiny, highly-branched microscopic tubes with a very large surface area which facilitates the diffusion of oxygen, carbon dioxide, water, nutrients and electrolytes through their walls. The internal pressures in the capillaries range from initial values of 25 mm Hg to approximately 10 mm Hg at their confluence on the venous side. The combined volume of the capillaries is small but their surface and cross-sectional areas are immense.

Collecting System. The collecting system which extends from the smallest venules to the largest terminal veins in the chest (vena cavae), conducts blood back to the heart. Veins are wide bored, large capacity, very thin-walled cylindrical vessels; some have one-way valves which prevent reflux and thereby assist in the transport of blood back to the heart. Their internal pressure is low, ranging from about 10 mm Hg at the tissues to about zero at their entrance to the heart.

BLOOD

Formed Elements

Blood is essentially a two-phase fluid consisting of formed cellular elements suspended in a liquid medium, the plasma. The formed elements are red cells (erythrocytes), white cells (leukocytes) and platelets. If a blood sample from a normal adult is centrifuged in a graduated test tube of uniform bore, the relative volume of the packed red blood cells, termed "hematocrit," will be about 40 to 45% of the total, as shown by the height of the packed cell column (Fig. 1–3). Thus, the red cells occupy about 40 to 45% of the total volume of blood

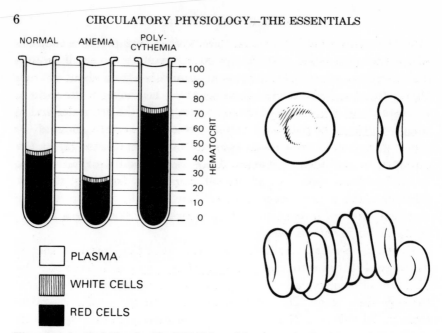

Figure 1-3. Red blood cells (RBC's) and hematocrit. Surface and cut views of red cells. RBC's sometimes gather into stacks called rouleaux which tend to offer increased resistance to flow. The percentage of packed RBC's in the centrifuged blood sample, termed the hematocrit, is increased in polycythemia and decreased in anemia. The corresponding changes in hemoglobin content alter the oxygen carrying capacity of the blood.

in the body. The white cells being less dense, will settle on top of the red cells in a thin so-called "buffy" layer. The remaining 55 to 60% is plasma, sometimes called the "plasmacrit."

The erythrocytes are biconcave discs about 2.4 μm in thickness and 8 μm in diameter which are produced in the bone marrow through a process known as erythropoiesis. Their biconcave shape increases the total surface area available for diffusion. The red cells owe their characteristic color to the presence of the pigment hemoglobin, which has a remarkable capacity to combine with and transport oxygen. In the normal adult there are about 4.5 to 5.5 million red blood cells per cubic millimeter of peripheral blood; a greater than normal red cell volume in the blood is called polycythemia. A deficiency of red blood cells is known as anemia which has physiological consequences because of the accompanying hemoglobin deficiency (Fig. 1–3).

In the normal individual, there are 5000 to 7000 white blood cells per cubic millimeter in the peripheral blood; an excess is usually termed leukocytosis and a deficiency, leukopenia. The white cells are mainly concerned with combating bacterial infections, with immune processes and with bodily defense. Platelets are vital elements for blood coagulation; there are about 150,000 to 300,000 platelets per cubic millimeter in peripheral blood but because of their small size (2–3 μm) they occupy only an insignificant fraction of the blood volume.

Plasma

The plasma or fluid fraction of the blood normally occupies about 55% of the blood volume and carries a variety of substances including plasma proteins (which are the major portion of the plasma solids), non-protein nitrogen, electrolytes, hormones, enzymes and blood gases. The normal concentrations of some of the more important constituents of plasma are given in Table 1-1.

Blood Volume

The total blood volume is the sum of the volume of the cells and plasma, both of which are usually determined by dilution methods.

Table 1-1. Normal Concentration of Plasma Constituents

	Per dl (deciliter) Plasma
Total protein	6.0 to 7.8 g
Albumin	3.2 to 4.5 g
Globulin	2.3 to 3.6 g
Fibrinogen	0.2 to 0.4 g
Glucose (fasting)	70 to 110 mg
Total lipids	400 to 1000 mg
Cholesterol	150 to 300 mg
Triglycerides	50 to 150 mg
Non-protein nitrogen (NPN)	20 to 45 mg
Blood urea nitrogen (BUN)	10 to 25 mg
Uric acid	3 to 7 mg
Creatinine	0.9 to 1.5 mg
Electrolytes (serum) Meq/L	
Na^+	136 to 145
K^+	3.5 to 5.0
Ca^{++}	4.5 to 5.5
Cl^-	98 to 110

This involves (in the case of plasma) the injection of an amount (A) of a test substance such as ^{125}I-labeled human serum albumin (HSA). After about a 10-minute mixing period, a sample of blood is withdrawn, the red cells removed by centrifugation and the plasma concentration (C) of the test substance determined. The total plasma volume (V) is then determined as: V (ml) $= A$ (mg)$/C$ (mg/ml).

The red blood cell volume can similarly be estimated with red cells labeled with radioactive chromium (^{51}Cr) using the same principle. The plasma volume, at any particular moment, represents a temporary balance between the intake of fluid and its output *via* kidneys, gastrointestinal tract *etc.*; while it may temporarily fluctuate over a period of time, in a relatively steady state, an individual's total blood volume usually remains remarkably constant. Since values in the normal adult generally range from 70 to 75 ml/kg of body weight, a 70-kg adult might therefore have a total blood volume of about 5000 ml with about 55% or 2750 ml of the total as plasma volume and about 45% or 2250 ml as total red cell mass.

The dilution principle assumes that none of the indicator material is lost and that perfect mixing occurs. This is not entirely true since some of the plasma protein (with indicator attached) is slowly eliminated during the test period and some ^{51}Cr is sequestered in the spleen and other reticuloendothelial organs. For more accurate determinations of cell and plasma volumes, the blood concentrations of the indicator material are followed over a 30- or 60-minute period, plotted against time on log graph paper and the original concentration estimated by extrapolating backward to zero time.

OXYGEN TRANSPORT

Although the assimilation and transport of oxygen is a definitive part of respiratory physiology, its importance to the normal and abnormal circulation warrants a brief review.

The chief constituent of the erythrocyte is hemoglobin (Hb), the primary oxygen carrier, which is normally present in a concentration of 14 to 15 g/dl of whole blood. Hb combines reversibly with oxygen to form oxyhemoglobin (HbO$_2$), the primary oxygen carrier. When exposed to certain drugs and other oxidizing agents, Hb is converted to a darker colored methemoglobin, which is present in only very small amounts in normal blood. Hb has a high affinity for carbon monoxide which can displace the O$_2$ to form carboxyhemoglobin; exposure to excessive amounts of carbon monoxide can significantly reduce the oxygen carrying capacity of the blood.

If blood is exposed to a sufficiently high oxygen pressure so that all the Hb is combined with oxygen to form HbO_2, it is "fully saturated"; under these circumstances, 1 g of Hb can combine with 1.39 ml of oxygen so that blood with a Hb concentration of 15 g/dl will then have an "oxygen capacity" of 20.8 ml/dl of blood or 20.8 vol %. The amount of oxygen with which each unit of Hb will actually combine is dependent primarily on the partial pressure of oxygen (Po_2) to which the Hb is exposed; this relationship is defined by the oxygen dissociation curve (Fig. 1–4).

In the alveoli of the lungs, where the Po_2 is normally at a high level, the blood will be about 97% saturated, that is, 97% of Hb is combined

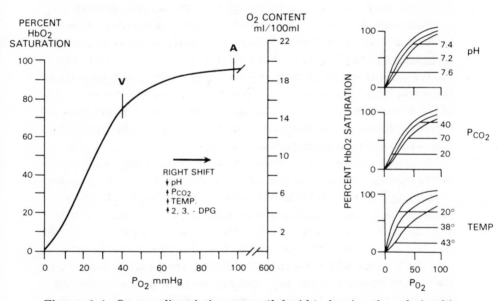

Figure 1-4. Oxygen dissociation curve (*left side*) showing the relationship between the partial pressure of oxygen (Po_2) and the percentage of oxyhemoglobin (HbO_2) saturation of the blood. In the alveoli of the lungs (*A*) the Po_2 is about 100 mm Hg which results in a 97% HbO_2 saturation. In the mixed venous blood returning from the tissues, the Po_2 has fallen to about 40 mm Hg and the HbO_2 saturation is approximately 75% (*V*). Small shifts of the curve to the right, which occur in the tissues because of the lower pH, higher Pco_2 and higher temperature, tend to lessen the affinity of Hb for oxygen and assist in release of oxygen to the tissues. (Adapted from J. B. West, *Respiratory Physiology*, p. 75. Baltimore: Williams & Wilkins Co., 1974.)

with O_2 (A in Fig. 1–4); in this case arterial blood with a Hb concentration of 15 g/dl will have an oxygen content of 20.2 ml/dl. After the blood has given up some of its oxygen in the tissues and reached the large veins (mixed venous blood) its Po_2 value will have decreased to about 40 mm Hg. As indicated in Figure 1–4, V, at this Po_2 the blood will be only about 75% saturated with oxygen and the blood oxygen content will be about 16 ml/dl; it can be seen that this blood will have released to the tissues about 4 ml of gaseous oxygen for each 100 ml of blood flow through the capillaries.

While oxygen content is determined primarily by the Po_2, it is also influenced to a lesser extent by four other factors, $i.e.,$ pH, Pco_2, blood temperature and the concentration of 2,3-diphosphoglycerate (2,3-DPG). An increased red cell concentration of the organic phosphate, 2,3-DPG, may occur in chronic hypoxia or chronic lung disease.

A decrease in pH or an increase in any of the other three will produce a "shift to the right" in the oxyhemoglobin dissociation curve (Fig. 1–4); the result is that at the same Po_2, less O_2 will be bound to the Hb and consequently more released to the tissues so that, in effect, there will be a lesser affinity of Hb for O_2. Conversely, an increase in pH or a decrease in Pco_2, blood temperature or 2,3-DPG will have the opposite effect, $i.e.,$ the dissociation curve will shift to the left, so there is greater affinity of hemoglobin for oxygen.

The shape of the oxygen dissociation curve has other implications; at the upper "plateau" portion of the curve where it is flatter, large changes in Po_2 will have relatively little effect on HbO_2 saturation and content. As a result, moderate decreases in Po_2 encountered at high altitude or other low oxygen environments result in smaller reductions in HbO_2 saturation and content than would ordinarily be the case, so that the hypoxia will be partially "buffered." On the other hand, in the capillaries, where the Po_2 falls sharply, as represented by the steep portion of the curve, the tissues have the advantage of being able to pick up a large supply of oxygen with only a small decrease in Po_2.

VOLUME AND PRESSURE

Volume and Pressure Distribution

The most important physical characteristics of the circulation are volume, pressure and flow. Volume and volume-pressure relations comprise the *statics* of the system and define the basic qualities which distinguish important functional properties of arteries and veins. Pressure and flow relate to the moving stream of blood and so characterize the *dynamics* of the circulation.

In the circulatory system, the volume is unevenly distributed, with about two thirds on the venous side (Fig. 1-5). Because many of the large capacity vessels—particularly the systemic venous, pulmonary arterial and pulmonary venous—are in the chest, about half of the circulatory blood volume is in the thorax; here it serves as a ready reservoir for venous return and cardiac filling when the heart needs to increase its output. However, this thoracic or "central" blood volume, being at low pressure, is relatively easily dislocated; for example, upon moving into the upright posture from the horizontal, 500 to 700 ml of systemic venous blood—most of it from the "central blood volume"— ordinarily gravitates to the veins below the diaphragm, *i.e.,* to the abdomen, pelvis and lower extremities. Although this blood remains

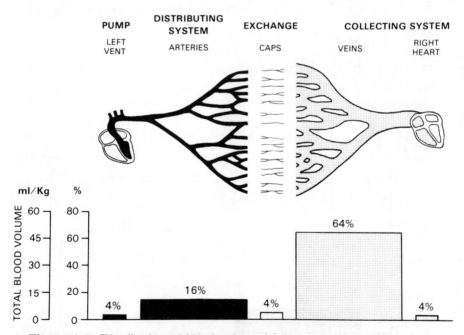

Figure 1-5. Distribution of blood volume in the systemic circulation. Not shown is the 8% fraction in the pulmonary vessels.

(at least temporarily) within the circulatory system, it is less readily available to the heart; its dislocation therefore reduces both the volume and the pressure of this central venous reservoir for cardiac filling. Thus upon standing, there is a temporary decrease in venous return and cardiac output of about 15 to 20%; this does not normally pose a circulatory problem but in certain cardiovascular disorders becomes a significant stress (Chapter 13).

Volume-Pressure Relations in Blood Vessels

Although about two thirds of blood volume is normally in the venous system and only about one sixth on the arterial side, the pressure distribution is quite different, being in almost inverse relation to the volume distribution (Fig. 1–6). This disposition of pressure and volume is due in large part to the structure and relative elasticity of the arteries and veins, that is, to their <u>pressure-volume relations</u>. While it is true that the entire arterial tree serves as a distributing conduit, all arteries are not alike; from an anatomical and functional standpoint

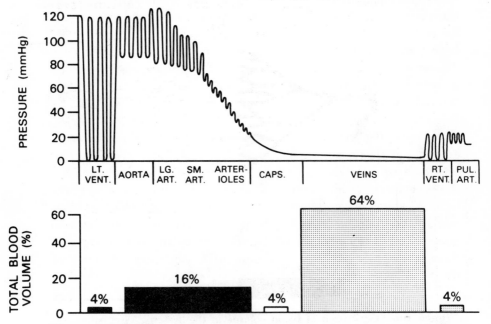

Figure 1-6. Pressure and volume distribution in the systemic circulation. Illustrating the inverse relationship between internal pressure and volume in different portions of the circulatory system.

they may be divided into two main groups which differ structurally and functionally from each other, and both of which, in turn, differ notably from veins.

1. Aorta and Large Arteries. All blood vessels have an endothelial lining and contain varying proportions of smooth muscle, elastin and collagen; however the aorta and the large arteries have unusually large amounts of elastin in their walls and thus are capable of considerable expansion and recoil. This quality enables them to store pressure energy as their walls are stretched during ventricular systolic ejection; with subsequent rebound of the vessel wall, this pressure energy can then be released as kinetic energy of flow in the succeeding diastole.

This helps to propel the blood toward the tissues during the diastolic phase of the cardiac cycle and promotes a more even flow to the capillaries. The large arteries are therefore the "pressure storers" of the circulation. As previously mentioned, the internal pressure in the large arteries is about 120/80 mm Hg.

2. Small Arteries and Arterioles. These vessels have fewer elastic fibers and more circular smooth muscle fibers. They have, therefore, contractile capabilities which, when activated, serve to constrict their lumen, dam back the flow, increase the pressure centrally (toward the heart), and decrease the pressure peripherally (toward the capillaries). These vessels thus serve as the "stopcocks" of the circulation and are usually called the "resistance" vessels. Their pressures generally range from about 60 to 90 mm Hg in the small arteries to about 40 to 60 mm Hg in the arterioles.

3. Veins. The veins are very thin-walled vessels with only small amounts of elastin and limited smooth muscle in their walls. Their pressures are low, ranging from about 10 mm Hg at the venular ends of the capillaries to about zero at the entrance of the vena cavae to the heart. Despite the fact that the venous system already holds four times more blood than the arterial system, if more fluid or blood is infused about 90% of the new fluid will be taken up by the veins because of their greater distensibility. As a consequence the veins are known as the "volume storers" of the circulation.

Distensibility and Compliance of Blood Vessels

In order to compare more precisely the volume and pressure characteristics of blood vessels, their "distensibility," that is, the increase in volume necessary to induce a unit pressure change, may be determined. If a large artery or vein is removed, tied at both ends and blood or fluid injected slowly into the lumen, the internal pressure will increase progressively as volume is added. If the percentage of volume change is plotted against the internal (transmural) pressure, pressure-volume or distensibility curves similar to those in Figure 1–7 will result.

The slope of the curve at any point (ratio of percentage of volume increase to pressure increase), which is a measure of the distensibility, varies with the degree of filling. The normal aorta has good distensibility and recoil at normal physiological pressures of about 75 to 150 mm Hg (Fig. 1–7A), which gives it the important property of a "pressure storer." However, at higher pressures such as 200 mm Hg,

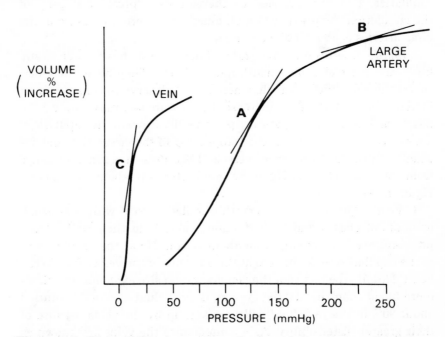

Figure 1-7. Distensibility (percentage of volume increase per unit pressure change) in a normal large artery and vein. Note the decreased slope of the arterial curve at higher pressure (*B*). Also the steep slope and much higher distensibility of the veins (*C*) at their physiological pressures (0–10 mm Hg) compared to the slope and distensibility of arteries (*A*) at their usual pressures (75–150 mm Hg).

when it is "overfilled," (Fig. 1–7*B*), its wall becomes more rigid and it has lesser distensibility, a smaller slope and less recoil.

In the latter case, the expandable qualities of elastin in the arterial wall are limited by relatively less expandable collagen and smooth muscle which, with stretching, reaches its limits and resists further distension. Distensibility is influenced, therefore, not only by the thickness and composition of the vessel wall but also by the degree of filling of the vessel.

As illustrated in Figure 1–7*C*, veins at their physiological pressures (0–10 mm Hg) have a high distensibility, ranging from five to six times that of arteries. However, vessels do not begin to show distensibility until they are filled. Since the veins have, in addition, about two to three times more volume than the arteries, the capacity of the venous system for storage of blood is about 12 to 18 times that of the arterial system and accounts for the primary function of veins as "volume storers" of the circulation.

"Compliance" and "capacitance," terms which are similar but not identical with distensibility, may be defined as the volume change per unit pressure change when fluid is added; these terms are commonly used to measure the expandability of vessels or of organ systems such as lungs. However compliance and capacitance have the disadvantage of defining the pressure-volume relationship without reference to the size of the vessel; obviously a given increment of volume will induce a much larger pressure rise in a smaller vessel than a large one so that the smaller vessel may have an apparently lesser compliance. For this reason "distensibility" or the *percentage* of volume change per unit of pressure, permits a more logical comparison of vessels of different sizes and types.

Distensibility may be altered by age, disease, autonomic stimulation and various drugs; in the elderly, the arterial walls become infiltrated with an increasing amount of less distensible fibrous tissue and so increase their stiffness (Fig. 1–8). This can affect pressure and flow relations in the entire arterial tree. This lesser distensibility at increased age is offset to some extent by the increased volume of the aorta in older individuals; the latter enables the aorta to accommodate the ejected left ventricular blood with less increase in pressure and thus with less expenditure of cardiac work than would ordinarily occur if aortic volume did not change.

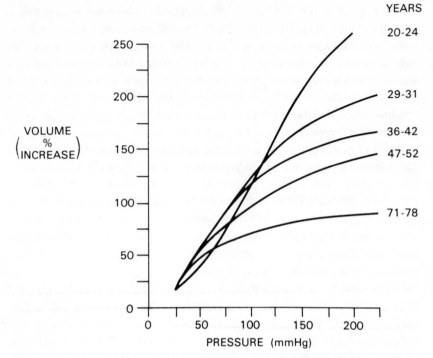

Figure 1-8. Decrease in aortic distensibility with advancing age. Note particularly the changes in distensibility within the physiological pressure range of 75 to 150 mm Hg. (From P. Hallock and J. C. Benson, *J. Clin. Invest.* 16:597, 1937.)

MEAN CIRCULATORY PRESSURE

As noted in Figure 1-6, the pressures in the circulatory system at rest in normal man range from a peak of 120 mm Hg at the aorta to about zero at the right atrium. If we consider the entire systemic circuit as a unit and sum all the pressure values and their respective volumes, what single mean pressure would represent the tendency to propel blood toward the heart? One way to determine this is to stop the heart momentarily and let the pressures equilibrate entirely on the basis of the volume within the system and the distensibility characteristics of the various parts of the circuit.

If this is done in an experimental animal whose pressures and volumes are comparable to an adult human, this equilibrated pressure or "mean circulatory pressure" in the systemic circuit is about 7 mm Hg. This rather low mean driving pressure is the result of the high percentage of blood in the low pressure venous system and the fact that the blood located in the high pressure arterial system will be displaced into the veins which have high distensibility. If after the cardiac arrest, the heart again begins to pump, it will again increase the pressure above this value on the arterial side and decrease it on the venous side.

This mean circulatory pressure, which is the net pressure gradient responsible for pushing blood toward the heart, will be further discussed in Chapter 7 with reference to factors influencing venous return and cardiac output in normal and abnormal situations.

TENSION IN THE BLOOD VESSEL WALL—LAPLACE'S THEOREM

In the preceding, consideration has been given to the internal volume and pressure of a blood vessel but not to the vessel wall itself, which obviously is a key factor. In a hollow, cylindrical tube, the circumferential tension, T, in the wall along the linear axis of a vessel is usually measured in dynes/cm and is calculated as the product of the transmural pressure, P_t (inside pressure minus outside pressure) and the radius, R (Fig. 1-9). This relationship (first defined by Laplace) was later expanded by Frank to include the factor of wall thickness "μ" as follows: $T = P_t R/\mu.$ This relationship suggests that in normal vessels in which the radius and wall thickness are in approximate proportion, the wall tension will vary with the transmural pressure and the two will tend to stay in reasonable balance. A capillary, for example, with a small radius and low pressure will require only a thin wall to sustain its lesser tension but a large artery with a greater pressure and radius will have a higher tension and a need for a thicker wall.

Wall tension may be important in certain pathological conditions such as severe arteriosclerotic disease in which an aortic wall may weaken, gradually bulge and become thinner at that point. With increasing radius and the progressive thinning, the tension at that site will further increase and the aorta may balloon and develop an "aneurysm" which might require surgical repair to prevent a rupture.

In congestive heart disease, the progressively increasing size of the failing heart may also produce inordinate tension in the wall of the heart. Since myocardial oxygen requirements are partly a function of myocardial tension, a reduction in heart size through medication will often promote increased cardiac efficiency by reducing wall tension

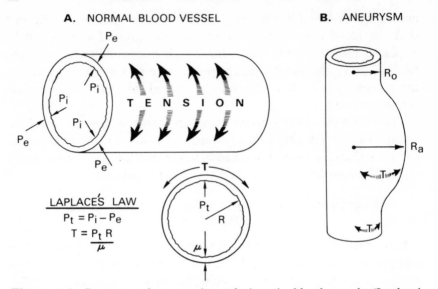

Figure 1-9. Pressure-volume-tension relations in blood vessels (Laplace's law). *A.* P_t, the transmural pressure (dynes/cm^2) is equal to the P_i (internal pressure) minus the P_e (external pressure). R is the radius (cm) and μ, the wall thickness (cm). T is the tension in the vessel wall (dynes/cm of longitudinal length). *B.* Aortic aneurysm is the atherosclerotic weakening of the vessel with resultant bulging. The increased radius R_a at the aneurysm site increases tension at that point and puts further stress on the aortic wall.

and, therefore, reducing the oxygen requirements per unit of mechanical work of the heart (see Chapter 14, Congestive Heart Failure).

REFERENCES

BADER, H.: Anatomy and physiology of vascular wall. In *Handbook of Physiology,* Section 2: *Circulation,* vol. II, ed. by W. F. Hamilton and P. Dow, pp. 865–889. Washington, D.C.: American Physiological Society, 1963.

BURTON, A. C.: *Physiology and Biophysics of the Circulation,* pp. 66–67, 119–120. Chicago: Year Book Medical Publishers, Inc., 1972.

GREEN, H. D.: Circulatory system: Physical principles. In *Medical Physics,* ed. by O. Glasser, pp. 228–251. Chicago: Year Book Medical Publishers, Inc., 1950.

HALLOCK, P., AND I. C. BENSON: Studies on the elastic properties of isolated human aorta. *J. Clin. Invest.* 16:595, 1937.

WEST, J. B.: *Respiratory Physiology,* pp. 72–88. Baltimore: Williams & Wilkins Co., 1974.

chapter 2

Hemodynamics

POISEUILLE'S LAW

In 1846, Poiseuille, a French physician, described the factors governing non-pulsatile flow of a homogeneous fluid through rigid tubes. He stated that if all other factors are held constant, the rate of flow, Q, through a cylindrical tube of length, L, and radius, r, was directly proportional to the driving pressure, ΔP (the difference in pressure between two ends of the tube), i.e., $Q \propto \Delta P$. In addition, Q was inversely proportional to the length of the tube, L, so $Q \propto 1/L$ and inversely proportional to the viscosity of the flowing liquid, η, $Q \propto 1/\eta$ and directly proportional to the fourth power of the radius of the tube, r, so that $Q \propto r^4$.

He added two necessary proportionality constants (π and 8) to elaborate "Poiseuille's law": $Q = \Delta P r^4 \pi / \eta L 8$.

Although blood is a non-homogeneous fluid, which in the body flows through branching, distensible tubes in a pulsatile manner, Poiseuille's law nonetheless gives good approximations and has proven very useful in understanding the *in vivo* circulation. Furthermore most of the factors in his equation are analogous to an ordinary hydraulic system and lend themselves to simplifications which may profitably be applied to basic and clinical cardiovascular problems.

RESISTANCE TO FLOW

If ΔP in Poiseuille's equation is considered to be the driving pressure, the remaining factors, $r^4 / \eta L$ may be considered impediments to flow.

19

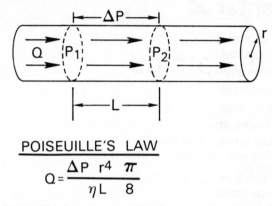

POISEUILLE'S LAW

$$Q = \frac{\Delta P}{\eta L} \frac{r^4}{8} \pi$$

Figure 2-1. Poiseuille's law. In an artificial system, flow through a cylindrical tube or any segment of a tube is directly proportional to ΔP, the driving pressure along the tube and the fourth power of the radius, and inversely proportional to the length of the segment and the viscosity of the liquid. $\pi/8$ is the proportionality constant.

← resistance

If these residual factors are collected together, inverted $\left[\dfrac{\eta L}{r^4} \right]$ and designated R, as resistance to flow, the formula can then be simplified to: Q (flow) = ΔP(driving pressure)$/R$ (resistance to flow), and by transposing: R (resistance to flow) = ΔP (driving pressure)$/Q$ (flow).

In this very basic and useful hemodynamic generalization, R is defined as that resistance provided by a vessel or circulatory bed, which permits a given pressure differential to produce a unit flow. It will be recalled that this equation is an analogue of Ohm's law, which states that with direct current, the electrical resistance, R (in ohms), is the ratio of electromotive force (in volts) and the current (in amperes).

By generalizing from an isolated cylindrical tube to the intact circulation in an organ or in the entire circulatory system, the vascular resistance to flow may similarly be estimated as the ratio of the pressure gradient across the organ or system and the blood flow through it. When this method of calculation is used, resistance is sometimes expressed in PRU units (pressure-resistance units) which are defined as mm Hg/ml of flow/min; an adult human, for example, with a mean aortic pressure of 100 mm Hg and a mean right atrial pressure of zero, would have a pressure gradient across the systemic circulation of 100 mm Hg (ΔP). If the cardiac output were 5 L/min, the total peripheral resistance (TPR) of the system would be: TPR = 100 mm Hg/5000 ml/min or 0.02 mm Hg/ml/min or 0.02 PRU units.

Although the concept of vascular resistance is commonly employed in basic cardiovascular studies, its clinical application has been somewhat limited because measurements of flow, particularly in individual organs and tissues, are still technically rather difficult.

In comparing vascular resistances of different organs and organisms, it should be noted that blood flow (the denominator) is strongly influenced by the size and vascularity of the organ while arterial pressure (the numerator) is not. Thus an infant with a body weight and cardiac output only $\frac{1}{20}$ that of an adult will have a calculated total vascular resistance much greater than the adult even though the relative dimensions of vessels and tissues as well as flow per unit mass may be generally similar. For this reason, when comparing organisms, vascular resistance is usually expressed on a weight basis, *e.g.*, per 100 g of tissue.

Components of Vascular Resistance

In the previous discussion of Poiseuille's law, the question of what actually constitutes resistance was temporarily bypassed. In transposing Poiseuille's law, the vascular resistance became $R = \eta L/r^4$.

It is seen that η, the viscosity, is the fluid resistance factor and L/r^4 the blood vessel resistance factor. While it seems reasonable that the viscosity and length of the system would be important in determining resistance to flow, the disproportionate role of the radius—which makes it the predominant factor in the equation—is rather surprising. The fourth power effect is due to the fact that flow in a cylinder is proportional, not to the radius of the tube, but to its cross-sectional area, which is an r^2 factor ($A = \pi r^2$); in addition, flow is a function of the velocity of the moving column, which in turn is proportional to the square of the distance from the axis to the vessel wall. The combination of these two r^2 terms and the consequent magnification of the radius factor has important implications for the control of flow in the intact organism.

Within the same vascular bed over a short period of time, neither length of the circuit nor blood viscosity would ordinarily change

① appreciably; the most important adjustment of vascular resistance, therefore, is accomplished by alteration of vessel diameter. A decrease in lumen diameter is brought about by contraction of the smooth muscle of the vessel wall, primarily of arterioles (vasoconstriction) which increases resistance to flow, or by relaxation of the tone of the muscle (vasodilation) which increases the lumen size and, therefore, decreases resistance. Thus, alteration of vascular resistance to an organ is almost entirely a function of the adjustment of the caliber of blood vessels; by virtue of the radius effect, large changes in resistance to flow can be brought about quickly with small changes in vessel diameter.

② Another way in which vascular resistance may be affected is by opening or closing of sections of capillary bed by constriction or relaxation of the precapillary sphincters. An example of this is skeletal muscle in which only about $\frac{1}{10}$ of the total capillary bed is open at rest; during exercise these sphincters open widely permitting a very large flow at low resistance. The effect is analogous to that which occurs with arteriolar dilation except that the resistance changes in the capillaries would generally be smaller because the pressure gradients along capillaries are much less than along arterioles. After we calculate TPR, as described above, how can we calculate the R of a part of the circuit, *i.e.,* determine the distribution of the resistance? If we assume a constant flow through all the collective cross sections of the entire circulation (Fig. 2-2), and if $R = \Delta P/Q$, the greatest resistance will lie in that segment in which the pressure fall is the greatest (*i.e.,* the arterioles) and the resistance is least where the pressure fall is least (*i.e.,* the aorta) (Fig. 2-2). The fact that the arterioles offer much greater resistance than the large arteries in spite of the more extensive cross-sectional area of the arteriolar bed (Fig. 2-6) is further evidence of the disproportionate resistance effect of the smaller radii on flow.

Series and Parallel Resistances

In a manner analogous to electrical circuits, vascular resistances may be in series or parallel (Fig. 2-3). If in series, the resistances are additive, but when in parallel they are additive as reciprocals so that $1/R_T = 1/R_1 + 1/R_2 + 1/R_3$ *etc.* This means that in a parallel circuit, R_T is less than any of the individual R terms.

Viewed as a total system, the large majority of the vascular resist-

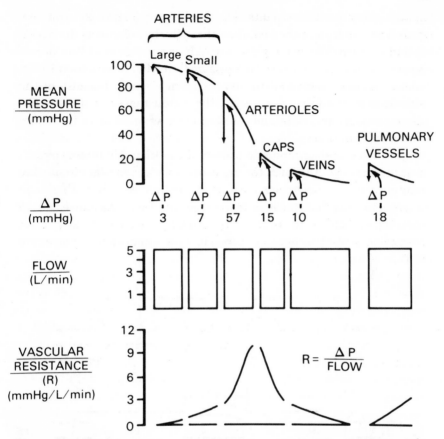

Figure 2-2. Vascular resistances in different segments of the circulation. The pressure fall (ΔP) is shown in different parts of the circulation (*top*) and is greatest at the arteriolar level. If the ΔP values (*2nd from top*) are divided by the flow, which is constant through all the segments (*3rd from top*), the vascular resistances of the different segments (*bottom*) can be estimated. It is highest at the arteriolar level.

ances of the organs and tissues of the body are in parallel. For the circulatory system this provides a significant advantage, not only because greater flow can be achieved with small changes of pressure but also because parallel vascular circuits permit greater flexibility in the control of flow to individual beds. Thus through manipulation of resistances, flow through one circuit can be increased or decreased without necessarily affecting the proximal arterial pressure or flow through other parallel circuits. For example, in Figure 2-3 (parallel resistances), if R_1 is increased, flow through that circuit is decreased without affecting the driving pressure ΔP or the resultant flow across circuits 2 and 3. By contrast, increase in R_1 in the series conduit (Fig. 2-3) will reduce flow to all the downstream circuits. Because of the awkwardness of adding reciprocals, the conductances of parallel circuits ($G = 1/R$) are sometimes used in place of resistances for hemodynamic calculations.

Figure 2-4 is a diagrammatic sketch of the main circulatory resistances of the body. Although the great majority of vascular circuits are in parallel, in certain organs such as the kidney and liver, the blood traverses two capillary beds in tandem so that their resistances are in series. The result of this is that the second capillary bed has a lower pressure and lesser ability to increase its flow when such increases are needed.

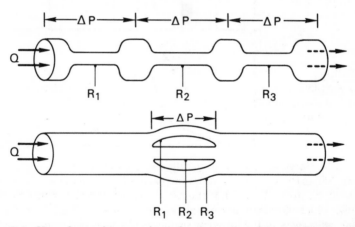

Figure 2-3. Vascular resistances in series (*upper*) and in parallel (*lower*). If across each series resistance (*upper*), the driving pressure, (ΔP), is 3 mm and the flow (Q) 1 ml/min, then each resistance (R) would be $\Delta P/Q$ or 3 mm Hg/ml/min and R_T (total resistance) = 9 mm Hg/ml/min. In parallel resistances, (*lower*) if across each resistance, the driving pressure (ΔP) were 3 mm Hg and the flow (Q) 1 ml/min, then the total resistance is calculated as $1/R_1 + 1/R_2 + 1/R_3$ or 1 mm Hg/ml/min. Note that when the three resistances are in parallel, the total resistance is only one ninth of that which would prevail if the three resistances were in series (*i.e.*, the ratio of $R_P/R_S = 1/9$) so that it takes a ΔP of only 1 mm Hg (instead of 9 mm Hg) to produce a flow of 1 ml/min.

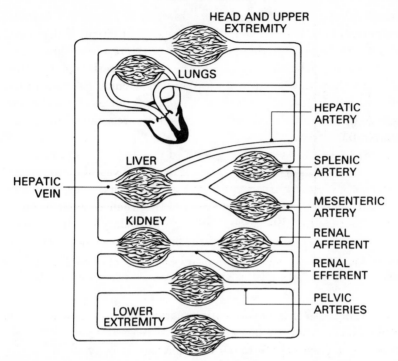

Figure 2-4. Diagrammatic sketch of vascular resistances in the body showing parallel and series circuits. Note the predominance of parallel circuits.

Viscosity

As indicated in Poiseuille's equation, the resistance to flow because of the friction of molecules in the moving stream is known as the viscosity. In a homogeneous liquid such as water in an artificial system, viscosity is a constant. However, in case of a two-phase medium such as blood flowing in an *in vivo* circulatory system, viscosity is not constant but depends on several factors: (a) the concentration of the suspended medium, *i.e.,* the cells; (b) the velocity of flow; and (c) the radius of the vessel.

If measured with reference to water, as is commonly done, the relative viscosity of plasma is about 1.3; the relative viscosity of whole blood depends mainly on the cell concentration or hematocrit as shown in Figure 2-5. At the usually prevailing hematocrit levels of about 42 to 45, the relative viscosity of blood is about 3.6 compared to water.

relative viscosity of blood 3.6
" " plasma 1.3

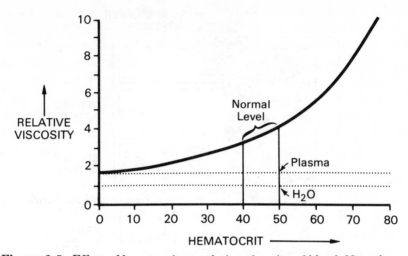

Figure 2-5. Effect of hematocrit on relative viscosity of blood. Note that as hematocrit increases, the relative viscosity increases disproportionately.

However, because of the exponential relationship, an increase of 10 in the hematocrit from the level of 40 will increase the viscosity about 25% and an increase of 20 (to 60) will increase viscosity about 60%.

In low hematocrit states such as anemia, viscosity and, therefore, vascular resistance both fall and as a result cardiac output rises. In high hematocrit conditions such as polycythemia and leukemia in which hematocrit levels may reach 60 to 70%, there is often a profound increase in systemic and pulmonary vascular resistance with the resultant elevation of blood pressures.

Two additional factors affect blood viscosity in a two-phase medium, namely, vessel bore and the flow rate. In tubes less than 200 μm in diameter—which would include arterioles, capillaries and venules—the relative viscosity of the blood decreases and offers less resistance to flow; this phenomenon, for which there is no satisfactory explanation, is sometimes called the Fåhraeus-Lindqvist effect.

A further peculiarity of two-phase fluids such as blood, is that at low flow rates, the apparent viscosity increases (anomalous viscosity); this phenomenon has been attributed to the disposition of red cells in the flowing stream; at higher velocities the cells accumulate in the axial part of the stream but at low velocities assume a more even distribution and hence offer greater flow resistance. Another factor that is probably involved in anomalous viscosity is the tendency of erythrocytes, at lesser flow velocities, to aggregate into stacks or "rouleaux" (Fig. 1-3). This effect has been found by some investigators to be exaggerated in low flow states such as burns or shock, causing pronounced cell clumping or "sludge" in the microcirculation with severe hindrance to flow and a resultant ischemia of the tissue.

It should also be mentioned that in the capillary bed, the blood hematocrit is usually about 10% less than in the large vessels for reasons which are not well understood at present.

It is evident, therefore, that in different parts of the circulation, there will be significant variations in vessel diameter, flow velocity and hematocrit and that the net effect on viscosity is not always predictable. Present evidence suggests, however, the hematocrit effect on viscosity is the most important and predominant one.

Under special circumstances, temperature may affect blood viscosity in a significant manner. There is about a 2% rise in viscosity per 1°C fall in temperature. During prolonged exposure to cold and high wind, the extremities may become chilled and the reduced flow effect of vasoconstriction will be enhanced by the shift of the HbO_2 dissociation curve to the left (Fig. 1-4); the added effect of increased blood viscosity may intensify the ischemia and increase the possibility of frostbite and serious damage to the part.

FLOW VELOCITY AND TURBULENCE

The linear velocity of blood flow varies widely in the circulatory system—from a mean value of about 30 to 35 cm/sec in the aorta to about 0.2 to 0.3 mm/sec in the capillaries as illustrated in Figure 2-6. If we assume that equal volumes will be transported through the different segments of the circulation in equal times, the mean flow velocity ($\bar{V}$) will vary inversely with the cross-sectional area; i.e., $\bar{V}$ (mm/sec) = flow (ml/sec)/cross-sectional area (πr^2 in mm^2).

By transposing the factors in the above equation, the circulation time (CT) between two points (A and B) in a closed circulation can be calculated as the quotient of the volume contained between A and B and the mean rate of flow between the two points, i.e., CT in sec = volume (A to B) in ml/mean flow (A to B) in ml/sec. In states of circulatory failure, an increased CT for the systemic circulation is

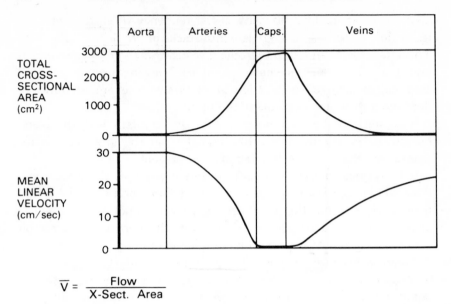

$$\overline{V} = \frac{Flow}{X\text{-Sect. Area}}$$

Figure 2-6. Relation of cross-sectional area and mean velocity of flow in the systemic circulation.

usually an index of decreased total flow, *i.e.*, of low cardiac output and inadequate circulation.

Poiseuille's law assumes that the different layers of molecules move parallel to each other in longitudinal streamlines, somewhat resembling concentric sleeves. The molecules adjacent to the vessel wall are stationary; each succeeding layer has increasing velocity with the maximum at the axis. Under these circumstances of "streamline" flow, the frictional resistance is independent of the pressure-flow relations and thus in the case of a homogeneous fluid is linear as has been previously described.

However, under certain circumstances, particularly at high velocities, the flow is no longer streamline but becomes turbulent with swirls and eddies (Fig. 2-7). In this case flow is approximately proportional to the square root of the pressure gradient rather than the pressure itself; there is, therefore, considerable increase in resistance now offered by the turbulent stream.

Reynolds has defined the factors affecting this phenomenon and stated that turbulence is likely to occur in a moving stream when the

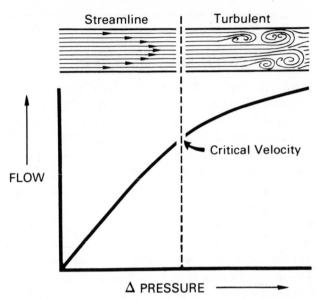

Figure 2-7. Relationship between velocity of flow and turbulence. (From T. C. Ruch and H. D. Patton, *Physiology and Biophysics,* Philadelphia: W. B. Saunders Co., 1974.)

Reynolds ratio (R_e) exceeds a value of about 1000 for blood or 2000 for homogeneous fluids: $R_e = \sigma \times v \times D/\eta$ in which σ is the density of the fluid (g/cm^3), v is the average velocity (cm/sec), D is the diameter of the vessel (cm) and η is the fluid viscosity (g/sec/cm^2). Since blood density is relatively constant, the factors tending to increase the Reynolds number and cause it to exceed the R_e are <u>increased velocity</u> of flow (such as in larger blood vessels), <u>decrease in viscosity</u> such as in anemia, and a <u>decrease in radius</u> of the vessel such as a stenosis (fixation) of a heart valve or coarctation (fibrotic constriction) of a blood vessel such as the aorta.

From the clinical standpoint, an important factor is that streamline flow is silent but <u>turbulence produces noise</u> which can often be heard with the unaided ear or with a stethoscope. Sounds used in the conventional determination of arterial blood pressure are audible because of the turbulence induced in the flow stream. In circulatory disease, defects in valves and constrictions of orifices will produce additional abnormal sounds which are used in clinical diagnosis (Chapter 3).

PRESSURE-FLOW CURVES

The vascular resistance of an organ, tissue or entire organism is determined—as has been discussed—mainly by the calibre of the blood vessels, particularly the arterioles. The calibre of the arterioles is determined by the "tonus" or contraction state of the vascular smooth muscle; the tone of the vascular muscle is, in turn, the result of a balance between the inherent tone due to the muscle itself, the sympathetic efferent vasoconstrictor impulses to the vessel and the dilator effect of local metabolites (Chapter 9).

In certain experimental and clinical situations, it is advantageous to measure peripheral vascular resistance. In the treatment of hypertension, *e.g.*, it is useful to know whether the high arterial pressure is due to excess vascular resistance or increased cardiac output. In peripheral vascular disease it would be helpful to quantify periodically the degree of vascular resistance of the region in order to follow the course of the disease or the effectiveness of various types of therapy. In the development of new vasoactive drugs, it is important to assess the ability of the drugs to produce or reverse a state of vasoconstriction; for these reasons, attempts are often made to determine the pressure-flow relations of an organ, tissue or entire circulatory system.

If, in an artificial system, a homogeneous fluid is perfused through a rigid tube and the radius and length of the cylinder and the fluid viscosity kept constant, the flow as predicted by Poiseuille's law will vary directly with the pressure gradient ΔP, so that a straight line relationship will result (Fig. 2-8). However, if the tube is distensible, the radius of the vessel will increase as the perfusion and the transmural pressure increase; the resultant flow will then increase according to the fourth power of the radius.

With *in vivo* systems, resistance to flow will be influenced not only by the distensibility of the vessels but also, as previously discussed, by the effect of vessel calibre and flow velocity. Flow resistance is also influenced by the type of tissue involved. In lung or skin tissue, for example, if perfusion rates are altered gradually rather than abruptly so that the vessels are permitted to adapt, a pressure-flow curve similar to that shown in Figure 2-9*a* will result.

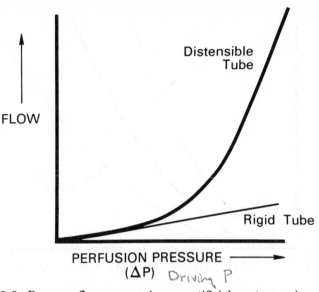

Figure 2-8. Pressure-flow curves in an artificial system using rigid and distensible tubes. Note that with increase in perfusion pressure, there is a large increase in flow in the distensible tube.

In the normal resting tissue (Fig. 2-9a) the curve is exponential and convex to the pressure axis; thus the flow through the tissue rises disproportionately with increasing perfusion pressure (ΔP) due mainly to the increased distension of the vessels as described above. This is a "passive" type of pressure-flow curve. In other tissues which show "autoregulation" the pressure-flow curve will have a different configuration (Chapter 9).

A pressure-flow perfusion system similar to this is frequently used to test the pharmacological effects of drugs on vascular smooth muscle. Injection of a constrictor agent such as norepinephrine will reduce the calibre of vessels and shift the curve to the right (Fig. 2-9c), *i.e.*, there will be less flow per unit pressure and the resistance of the bed will be increased. Similarly if a vasodilating drug such as histamine is injected (Fig. 2-9d) there will be a reduction in the pressure-flow ratio and lesser resistance to flow.

It will be noted that these pressure-flow curves do not go through the origin, that is, flow goes to zero while there is still positive pressure

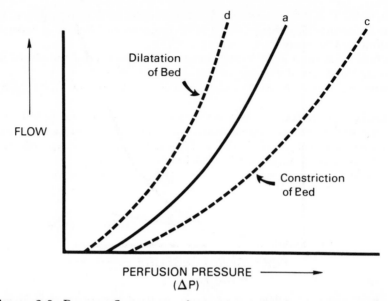

Figure 2-9. Pressure-flow curve of cutaneous vascular bed. As perfusion pressure is increased, the flow to the vascular bed increases disproportionately, *i.e.*, the peripheral resistance decreases. If a vasoconstrictor drug is injected, the pressure-flow curve changes from *a* to *c* indicating a general increase in vascular resistance. After a vasodilator drug, the pressure-flow curve will resemble that shown at *d*.

in the perfusion system. The reason for this phenomenon, which occurs in certain tissues, is not known; one theory is that as the vascular smooth muscle contracts, its inherent constrictive force and the resultant tension of the wall become greater than the distending force of the internal pressure; as the lumen becomes smaller, the tension becomes disproportionately greater than the distending pressure and the tension "wins," closing the vessel before the pressure has dropped to zero. The internal pressure which still exists when the vessel closes is known as the "critical closing pressure." Regardless of the explanation, the phenomenon is a potential hazard in low flow states such as shock in which tissues already ischemic are further threatened with sudden complete cessation of flow to certain capillary beds.

REFERENCES

BURTON, A. C.: *Physiology and Biophysics of the Circulation.* Chicago: Year Book Medical Publishers, Inc., 1972.

CARO, C. G., T. J. PEDLEY, AND W. A. SEED: Mechanics of the circulation. In *Cardiovascular Physiology,* vol. 1, *MTP International Review of Science.* Baltimore: University Park Press, 1974.

COULTER, N. A., AND J. R. PAPPENHEIMER: Development of turbulence in flowing blood. *Am. J. Physiol.* 159:401–408, 1949.

FOLKOW, B., AND E. NEIL: *Circulation.* London: Oxford University Press, 1971.

GREEN, H. D., C. A. RAPELA, AND M. C. CONRAD: Resistance and capacitance phenomena in terminal vascular beds. In *Handbook of Physiology,* Section 2: *Circulation,* vol. II, ed. by W. F. Hamilton and P. Dow, pp. 935–960. Washington, D.C.: American Physiological Society, 1963.

TAYLOR, M. G.: Hemodynamics. *Annu. Rev. Physiol.* 35:87–116, 1973.

chapter 3

The Heart: Structure and Function

FUNCTIONAL ANATOMY

The atria, whose walls consist mainly of two thin, overlying muscular sheaths arranged at right angles to each other, serve as blood reservoirs as well as pumps. The two thicker-walled ventricles pump blood from the low-pressure venous systems into the higher-pressure arterial systems.

In the pulmonary circuit, the right ventricle receives venous blood at about zero pressure and propels it into the pulmonary artery to a peak systolic pressure of about 25 mm Hg. The blood is oxygenated in the pulmonary capillaries and returned to the left heart. The left ventricle takes oxygenated blood, again at about zero pressure, and pumps it at a peak pressure of about 120 mm Hg into the aorta and systemic circuit and then to all the tissues of the body. The pulmonary circuit, because of its lower pressure and its shorter, wider-bore vessels with thinner walls, is characterized as a low-pressure, low-resistance system.

$$W_p = SV \times P_{\overline{ma}}$$

The ventricles generate pressure energy by ejecting blood against arterial resistance, and kinetic energy by imparting velocity to the blood. Pressure work—which usually comprises more than 95% of the mechanical energy expended by the heart—can be estimated as the product of the stroke volume and mean arterial pressure against which the ventricle works. Since the two ventricles eject similar volumes at identical heart rates, the left ventricle, because of its higher ejection pressure, performs about five to seven times as much pressure work as the right.

MYOCARDIAL CONTRACTION

The myocardial muscle of each ventricle consists of three interdigitating layers (Fig. 3-1). The two outer muscle layers are oriented obliquely from the base of the heart (superior portion), which is the area of attachment to the aorta and other great vessels, to the apex, which is the tapered, free portion. Upon contraction, the oblique fibers shorten the ventricular wall and pull the apex anteriorly and toward the base. The circumferential fibers constrict the ventricular diameter.

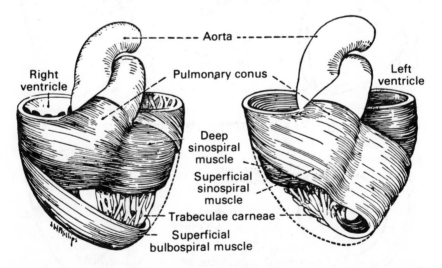

Figure 3-1. Components of the myocardium. The outer muscle layers pull the apex of the heart toward the base; the inner circumferential fibers constrict the lumen, particularly of the left ventricle. (From R. F. Rushmer, *Cardiovascular Dynamics*. Philadelphia: W. B. Saunders Co., 1976).

Right Ventricle

X-ray studies of the heart chambers have shown that the right ventricle has a concave outer wall and during contraction moves toward the interventricular septum with a bellows-like action, while the atrioventricular (AV) groove, or external depression, separating the right atrium and right ventricle, shortens toward the apex (Fig. 3-2). This anatomical configuration permits the thin and flexible wall of the right ventricle to eject a large volume of blood with a minimal amount of shortening against a low outflow pressure. However, if the pulmonary valve becomes thickened and stenotic, the resistance against which the right ventricle contracts will be much increased and flow into the pulmonary artery impeded; the right ventricular muscle then hypertrophies and may gradually approach the left ventricle in wall thickness.

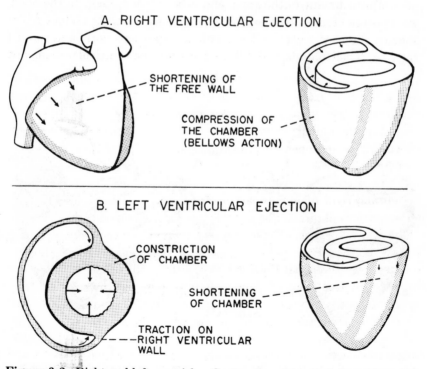

A. RIGHT VENTRICULAR EJECTION

SHORTENING OF
THE FREE WALL

COMPRESSION OF
THE CHAMBER
(BELLOWS ACTION)

B. LEFT VENTRICULAR EJECTION

CONSTRICTION
OF CHAMBER

SHORTENING
OF CHAMBER

TRACTION ON
RIGHT VENTRICULAR
WALL

Figure 3-2. Right and left ventricles. Contraction characteristics and modes of emptying. (From R. F. Rushmer, *Cardiovascular Dynamics.* Philadelphia: W. B. Saunders Co., 1970.)

Left Ventricle

As indicated above, left ventricular contraction involves both a decrease in diameter and a shortening of the axis between the base and apex of the heart; the net result is a movement of the mitral valve toward the apex. Simultaneously, the interaction of the various cardiac muscle groups produces a lifting effect on the apex, moving it toward the anterior chest wall and producing a palpable impulse at the left midclavicular line at about the interspace between the fifth and sixth ribs. The left ventricle with its more cylindrical outline (Fig. 3-2) has a mechanical advantage over the right ventricle in generating stroke volume and power, since the volume it ejects through a decrease in the diameter of a cylinder is a function of the square of the radius, rather than a linear function. The thick-walled and heavier left ventricle is also thought to provide a type of splint against which the outer wall of the right ventricle is pulled, thus ejecting the right ventricular blood by means of a squeezing, bellows-like action.

HEART VALVES

Efficient pumping action of the heart requires a minimum of reflux as the blood is transported. This is achieved through two sets of unidirectional, reciprocating valves. One pair, the aortic and pulmonic (also called semilunar) valves are located at the exits of the right and left ventricles and open and close passively. The three-cusped aortic valve (Fig. 3-3, *right*) when open, does not flatten against the aortic wall; this is important since it permits blood to flow unimpeded into the left and right main coronary arteries, whose openings are located in the aortic wall directly behind the open valve leaflets.

The two AV valves consist of the "tricuspid" on the right and the "mitral" on the left; these open toward the ventricles permitting blood to enter from the atria. Both valves are thin-walled and attached at the lower or free sides of their leaflets to papillary muscles on the ventricular walls by means of thin, stringy chordae tendineae (Fig. 3-3, *left*). The papillary muscles contract when the ventricles contract and so prevent the valves from bulging too far into the atrial chamber during ventricular contraction. A small amount of blood may occasionally regurgitate through a normal AV valve during ventricular contraction but with little effect on cardiac function; however, if one of the chordae tendinea becomes ruptured, the valve leaflet to which it

MITRAL VALVE

AORTIC VALVE

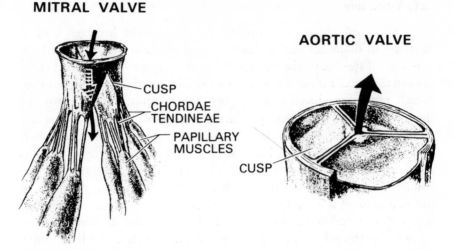

Figure 3-3. The mitral and aortic valves. The chordae tendineae and papillary muscles prevent the backward herniation of the mitral valve into the atrium during ventricular systole. (From A. C. Guyton, *Textbook of Medical Physiology*. Philadelphia: W. B. Saunders Co., 1976.)

is attached may bulge significantly, producing an incompetent valve with regurgitation of a sizable fraction of the blood backward into the atrium during ventricular systole with a marked loss of pumping efficiency. This complication, which may follow a "myocardial infarction" or "heart attack," may result in rapid death.

The AV valves have larger cross-sectional areas than the semilunar valves and are subjected to less mechanical force during valve opening and closure.

METHODS OF STUDYING CARDIAC FUNCTION

The pressure changes described in the following section are determined in the human subject with high-fidelity pressure transducers; these are attached to long, thin tubes (catheters) which are threaded into the heart chambers and the large vessels through a peripheral vein or artery (cardiac catheterization). If a radioopaque contrast material is injected, the outlines of the chambers can be visualized. With high speed fluoroscopy, rapid single or biplane photography, ultrasound and other techniques (Chapter 7), the rate of movement of the cardiac wall, the stroke volume and the emptying characteristics can be studied. These methods are used routinely in many cardiac catheterization laboratories. A more detailed description of methods for recording pressure and flow in the vascular system is given in Chapter 4 and for determination of cardiac output in Chapter 7.

For more precise study of heart sounds and murmurs, a small microphone is placed on the chest wall. The sound vibrations are amplified and recorded on an oscilloscope or polygraph; on the record, known as a *phonocardiogram,* the sounds appear as oscillations and through use of filters and other special devices, permit a more accurate analysis of sound frequency and intensity and their clinical significance.

An additional technique of great clinical value is the recording of the electrical changes generated by the heart, *i.e.,* the electrocardiogram (ECG). The development of multiple leads for more precise electrical recording at different points on the body has aided considerably in the diagnosis of certain cardiac disturbances such as arrhythmias. Electrical characteristics of the heart are described in Chapter 5.

THE CARDIAC CYCLE

The cardiac cycle embraces a combination of mechanical, electrical and valvular events whose interrelationship is complex but essential to the understanding of how the heart functions and how disease processes affect it. At rest, the normal adult heart beats at a rate of about 70 to 75 per minute. Blood flows from the atria to the ventricles and from the ventricles to the large arteries at a velocity which is determined by the pressure differences between the chambers. Normally the valves offer no resistance and open or close as a function of the relative pressures exerted by the flowing stream and the energy imparted by the contractions of the atrial and ventricular musculature.

At a rate of 75 per minute, the complete cycle for filling and emptying of the chamber would occupy 0.8 sec or 800 msec (Fig. 3-4). The cardiac cycle is divided into systole and diastole. Left ventricular systole, which is the contractile period of the left heart, extends from the early rise of ventricular pressure and the closure of the AV valve (Fig. 3-4A) to the closure of the aortic valve and the beginning of diastole (Fig. 3-4C). During most of the period from B to C, the ventricular pressure is higher than the aortic, the aortic valve is open and the ventricle ejects blood into the arterial system. At C the aortic valve closes.

Diastole, which is the period of ventricular relaxation and filling,

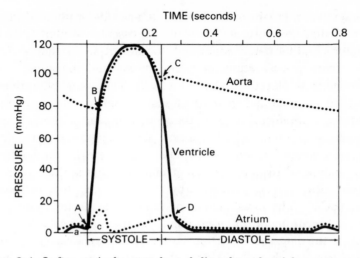

Figure 3-4. Left ventricular systole and diastole and atrial pressure waves. As the ventricle contracts at *A,* the mitral valve closes; as pressure increases and exceeds aortic, the aortic valve opens (*B*). As ejection is completed, the pressure falls below aortic and the aortic valve closes (*C*). As ventricular pressure falls below atrial, the mitral valve opens (*D*) and diastolic filling continues until the ventricle contracts again.

begins with the closing of the aortic valve (*C*); when the ventricular pressure falls below the atrial, the AV valve opens (*D*) and the ventricle begins to fill. Diastole ends when the ventricle again contracts and the new cycle begins.

At a heart rate of 75 per minute, systole will ordinarily occupy 250 to 300 msec; thus almost two thirds of the cycle (or about 500 to 550 msec) is taken up with diastolic filling. However, with an increase in heart rate up to 180 per minute, which can occur in severe exercise, the length of the total cycle is much reduced (to about 330 msec); most of the reduction is in diastolic time, which will ultimately restrict ventricular filling and limit cardiac output.

All cardiac events are normally timed according to systole and diastole of the ventricles, even though, as will be seen, this may not always coincide with the state of activity of other parts of the heart. Figure 3-4 and most of the subsequent figures refer, for reasons of illustration, only to the left ventricle; it should be emphasized that the events of the right side of the heart are analogous and that the right atrium and ventricle have similar timing of their electrical, mechanical and valvular events. The primary differences in the cardiac cycle between the two sides of the heart are those relating to the lower pressures in the right ventricle and pulmonary artery.

Role of the Atria

From a performance standpoint, the ventricles are necessarily the central factors in the cardiac cycle; the atria, however, play a significant supporting role. The normal atrial pressure curve has three positive deflections (Fig. 3-4). Shortly after the P wave of atrial depolarization (discussed below) the atria contract with a resulting positive _a wave_ which occurs late in diastole; when systole begins, the ventricular contraction causes a pressure wave to be transmitted through the thin-walled AV valves to the atria and also to the adjacent large veins resulting in the atrial _c wave_. During the last half of systole, as venous blood returns from the peripheral veins and the AV valves remain closed, atrial filling continues and atrial pressure rises with a resulting positive deflection called the _v wave_.

The atrial contraction, late in ventricular diastole, aids materially in conveying blood to the ventricle and may contribute as much as 25 to 30% of the total ventricular filling. In some disease states, in which atrial contraction is absent, the heart is usually able, over a period of time, to compensate for the loss of this atrial pump and can function reasonably well under resting conditions; however, during stress or in exercise, the absence of the atrial pump may result in a serious functional impairment of cardiac output with a resultant fatigue and other signs of acute heart failure.

Electrical Events of the Cycle

In order for the cardiac muscle to contract, there must be a preceding action potential which initiates the electrical and ionic events that culminate in ventricular systole. The ECG, which is recorded at the body surface, is a graphic representation of the summed voltage changes produced by electric depolarization and repolarization of the heart. These electrical impulses begin at the sinoatrial (SA) node in the right atrium, spread over the entire heart and initiate the contraction wave. The electrical phase of the cardiac cycle begins with excitation of the atrium, or atrial depolarization, which is denoted on the ECG by an initial upward deflection, a positive wave, called the P wave (Fig. 3-5); atrial contraction follows shortly thereafter.

After completion of the P wave, the ECG trace returns to base level, *i.e.,* isoelectric line. About 0.16 to 0.22 seconds following the onset of the P wave, there occur a series of waves, a negative Q wave preceding an R and a negative S following the R. This QRS complex is caused by electrical depolarization of the ventricles and is quickly followed by ventricular contraction. After a short interval, another deflection, the T wave, appears in the ECG which corresponds to repolarization of the ventricular muscle mass. The ECG then returns to the isoelectric line and usually there is electrical silence for the remainder of diastole.

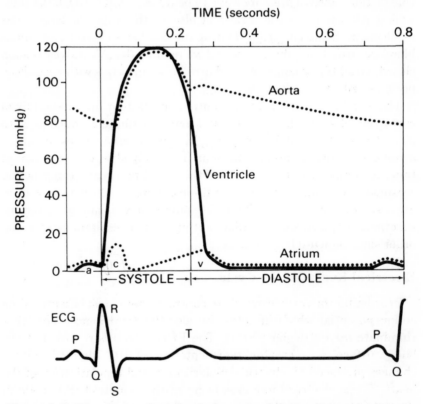

Figure 3-5. Electrical and mechanical events of the cardiac cycle. Showing the P wave (atrial depolarization) the QRS complex (ventricular depolarization) and the T wave (ventricular repolarization). Note that depolarization inevitably precedes the mechanical contraction.

The S-T segment is an important phase of the record because it is specifically distorted in myocardial ischemia.

It should be emphasized that the action potential is the indispensable forerunner to cardiac contraction. The heart has a spontaneous, intrinsic rhythmicity and automaticity, and contraction is inevitably coupled to excitation. Electrical characteristics of the heart are considered in greater detail in Chapter 5.

Ventricular Systole

It is necessary to examine more closely some of the events associated with the cardiac cycle. Systole is often divided into three parts—an *isovolumic contraction period, a rapid ejection period* and a *slower ejection period.*

Isovolumic (Isometric) Contraction Period (ICP). The ICP is an important interval between the closure of the mitral and the opening of the aortic valve, so called because there is no change in ventricular volume (Fig. 3-6); several significant events occur during this period. The rate of rise of ventricular pressure (dP/dt), which is sometimes used to characterize the contractile ability of the heart (Chapter 6), is maximum during this time. In addition, during the ICP, the atrial c wave occurs and the aortic and pulmonary arterial pressures are at their lowest level at this point, just before the opening of the aortic and pulmonary valves.

Rapid Ejection Period. The first one third of systole is comprised of the rapid ejection period, during which about two thirds of the ventricular volume is emptied into the aorta. Toward the end of this period, the aorta begins to distend as it absorbs the impact of the ejected blood and the rate of rise of aortic pressure decreases. The normal end-diastolic volume (EDV) is about 120 ml and the end-systolic volume (ESV) about 40 ml. Thus the average stroke volume (SV) is about 80 ml, and the ejection fraction (EF) about 67%. A decrease in EF is a common sign of a weakened myocardium.

Slower Ejection Period. At the peak of the aortic pressure curve, the ventricles begin to relax slightly and blood continues to flow from the ventricle to the aorta, but at a lesser rate—the slower ejection period. Near this point, the aortic pressure actually exceeds the left ventricular pressure by a few millimeters of mercury, but outflow continues because of the rapidly moving bolus of blood; with the

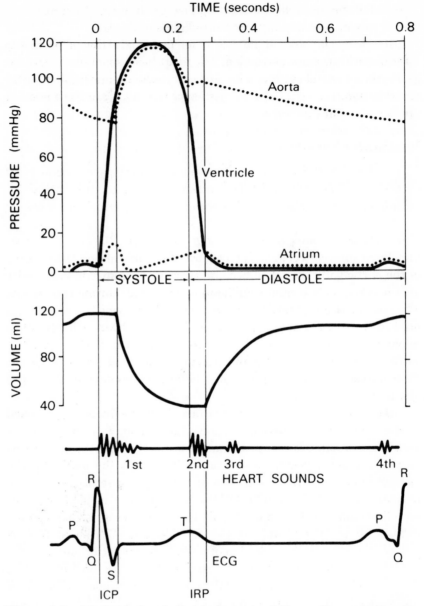

Figure 3-6. Mechanical and electrical events of the cardiac cycle showing also the ventricular volume curve and the heart sounds. Note the isovolumic contraction period (ICP) and the relaxation period (IRP) during which there is no change in ventricular volume because all valves are closed. The ventricle decreases in volume as it ejects its contents into the aorta. During the first third of systolic ejection—the rapid ejection period—the curve of emptying is steep.

reversal of the pressure gradient, the flow also reverses briefly and the aortic valve closes, producing the second heart sound.

Because the valves and aorta are distensible, they recoil, producing a secondary pressure wave in the aortic curve with a notch between the primary and secondary pressure curve which is referred to as the dicrotic notch. As these events occur in the left side of the heart, a similar sequence of events is occurring in the right ventricle and pulmonary artery and results in closure of the pulmonary valve.

In practice, the term systole is often referred to as the period between the beginning of the first and the beginning of the second heart sounds although clearly one may refer to atrial systole, right ventricular systole *etc.*

Ventricular Diastole

During the period between closing of the semilunar valves and the opening of the AV valves, *i.e.*, the isovolumic relaxation period (IRP), the ventricular pressure falls rapidly while the ventricular volume remains constant. When ventricular pressure falls below atrial pressure, the AV valves again open and the period of ventricular filling begins.

The ventricles become approximately two thirds filled within the first one third of ventricular diastole; this is referred to as the passive rapid-filling phase. In late diastole, ventricular filling is again augmented by atrial contraction; this is known as the active rapid-filling phase. The period between these two rapid-filling phases is sometimes called diastasis (a slower filling phase).

HEART SOUNDS

The two primary heart sounds are usually heard as a "lup-dup," a low pitched first sound, followed by a quicker, higher-pitched second. The intensity of heart sounds, as heard at the chest wall, depends upon several factors, *i.e.,* the rate of rise of ventricular pressure, the physical characteristics of the ventricles and valves, the volume contained in the heart, the position of the AV valve leaflets at the beginning of ventricular systole and the transmission characteristics of the chest wall. The relationship of the heart sounds to other events of the cardiac cycle is shown in Figure 3-6. The major components of the heart sounds are associated with the abrupt acceleration and deceleration of blood in and near the heart, but there is not full agreement on the relative significance of valve activity and muscle vibration.

The first heart sound (S₁) is associated with the closure of the mitral and tricuspid valves at the start of ventricular systole and the two components can sometimes be distinguished. If so, the first component of S_1 is mitral in origin and the second component, tricuspid.

The second heart sound (S₂) is usually of higher frequency and shorter duration than the first. It marks the end of ventricular systole and the beginning of diastole and is associated with the closure of the semilunar valves. It consists of two components, aortic and pulmonic. Normally, the aortic valve closes several milliseconds before the pulmonic and the time difference is accentuated during the inspiratory phase of respiration.

This respiratory delay in closing of the pulmonary valve produces a "physiological" splitting of the second heart sound and is mainly due to the sudden decrease in intrathoracic pressure associated with inspiration. This in turn, causes a temporary increase in venous return, and an increase in right heart volume; with the increased right ventricular output there is a temporary prolongation of ejection time and a delay in pulmonary valve closure. At the same time, pulmonary venous return to the left heart is diminished so that left ventricular stroke volume decreases and the aortic valve closes slightly earlier. Variations in the degree of splitting of the second heart sound occur in certain types of congenital heart disease and in cases of abnormal conduction of the electrical impulses of the heart.

A third heart sound (S₃), shown in Figure 3-6, is associated with the passive rapid-filling phase. For reasons which are not clear, a physiological third sound may be present in younger individuals; however, if it occurs after the age of 40 years, it is generally considered abnormal. It may occur in fever, cardiac failure and certain other cardiac disorders. *The fourth heart sound (S₄)* is associated with the active rapid-filling phase (Fig. 3-6). While it can often be recorded by phonocardiography, it is generally not audible. When it does occur, it is usually recorded at the peak of atrial contraction and may be associated with increased atrial pressures.

PATHOPHYSIOLOGY

Heart Murmurs

Disturbances of normal blood flow patterns in the heart and great vessels often result in abnormal sound vibrations in the auditory frequency ranges which are called murmurs. They are classified on the basis of their timing as systolic, diastolic and continuous murmurs. If the aortic or pulmonary valve is diseased or deformed, the increased turbulence through the narrowed or distorted orifice results in the crescendo-decresendo systolic murmur characteristic of aortic or pulmonary valve disease (Fig. 3-7 *I*).

If AV valve closure is incomplete because of disease of the mitral or tricuspid valves, the valve will become incompetent and blood will regurgitate into the atrium producing a blowing "whoosh" noise following the first heart sound. If this systolic murmur persists throughout systole, as indicated in Figure 3-7 *II,* it is sometimes referred to as a pansystolic or holosystolic murmur.

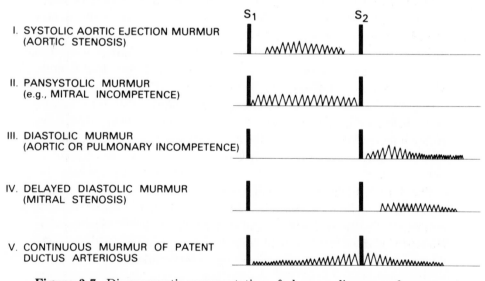

Figure 3-7. Diagrammatic representation of phonocardiograms of common systolic and diastolic murmurs. S_1 and S_2 = 1st and 2nd heart sounds. (Adapted from P. Wood, *Diseases of the Heart and Circulation,* 3rd ed., Philadelphia: J. B. Lippincott Co., 1968).

Abnormal heart sounds may also occur during diastole and are associated either with an abnormality of AV valve opening (usually mitral) or an abnormality of semilunar valve closure (usually aortic). A murmur originating at the aortic valve and heard in early diastole is produced by incomplete closure of the aortic valve at the end of systole. Such an abnormality may be due to fibrosis or stiffening of the valve in the open position or destruction of valve leaflets. The defect causes regurgitation of blood back into the left ventricle at the end of systole through the incompetent valve, producing the diastolic murmur of aortic regurgitation or aortic insufficiency (Fig. 3-7 *III*).

Stenosis of the mitral valve may cause abnormal heart sounds during early or late diastole, as shown in Figure 3-7 *IV*. The early component of this murmur is often initiated with an opening snap of the mitral valve; the late component may be associated with the atrial systole, just before the onset of ventricular systole, and is referred to as a "presystolic" murmur. See also the following section for a further description of aortic stenosis.

In addition to the preceding, certain types of murmurs may be heard throughout systole and diastole, such as the murmur of the patent ductus arteriosus (Figure 3-7 *V*); a constant movement of blood through the patent ductus will occur during the entire cycle and produce a heart murmur with a continuous machinery-like quality, with a waxing and waning of intensity. Blood flow is continuous through the patent ductus arteriosus during the entire cycle because of a persistent pressure gradient from the aorta to the pulmonary artery during both systole and diastole. (This will not occur if there is a reversal in the pressure gradient due to severe pulmonary hypertension.)

The fourth heart sound, when present, usually indicates a non-compliant ventricle; it commonly occurs in ischemic heart disease, pulmonic or aortic stenosis and pulmonary and systemic hypertension. However, it does not occur in mitral or tricuspid stenosis since the sound is also dependent upon rapid ventricular inflow.

Abnormal Intracardiac Pressures and Oxygen Saturations

In the preceding chapters, it has been pointed out that the circulation is maintained on the basis of pressure, flow and oxygen gradients and normal values in different parts of the circulatory system have been cited. There are, however, variations in the healthy population and even wider variations in disease.

In the following section are given approximate ranges of normal cardiac pressures and oxygen saturations; two examples are also presented to illustrate how deviations in these normal relations may be produced by cardiac disorders. In later chapters the effects of other vascular diseases will be considered more fully.

While there are phasic changes, mean right atrial pressure in the normal adult varies from about 0 to 6 mm Hg, right ventricular systolic pressure from 25 to 30 mm Hg, and diastolic pressure from 0 to 5 mm Hg. In the pulmonary artery, systolic pressure varies from about 22 to 30 mm Hg and diastolic pressure from about 9 to 12 mm Hg.

The left atrium shows pulsatile fluctuations similar to the right, but with slightly higher mean values ranging from about 4 to 10 mm Hg. Left ventricular pressure ranges from about 120 to 140 mm Hg systolic, and from 0 to 10 mm Hg diastolic. Aortic systolic pressures vary in the young adult from about 120 to 140 mm Hg and diastolic pressures from about 70 to 80 mm Hg.

In *aortic stenosis* there is an obstruction to left ventricular ejection which produces an increased systolic pressure gradient between the left ventricle and aorta (Fig. 3-8, *lower*). In an effort to maintain adequate flow, the left ventricular systolic pressure begins to rise and may increase to levels above 200 mm Hg with an aortic systolic pressure of 100 mm Hg or less. With progressive stenosis, this abnormal ventricular-aortic pressure gradient (Fig. 3-8, *lower*) requires an increased pressure work and may result in severe left ventricular hypertrophy (Chapter 15). However in spite of this hypertrophy, the insufficient output due to the stenosis and inadequate coronary perfusion for the enlarged ventricle results in cardiac failure.

Oxygen Concentrations in the Cardiac Chambers. In the vena cavae, right atrium, right ventricle and pulmonary artery, the blood oxygen content is about 15 to 16 ml/dl of blood and the oxygen saturation is normally 70 to 80%. Usually there is a slight decrease in oxygen saturation at the level of the right atrium where blood from the coronary sinus with a very low oxygen content and saturation mixes with blood from the vena cava. On leaving the pulmonary capillary bed the blood is usually 97 or 98% saturated with an oxygen content of 19 to 20 ml/dl blood. Because of drainage into the left heart

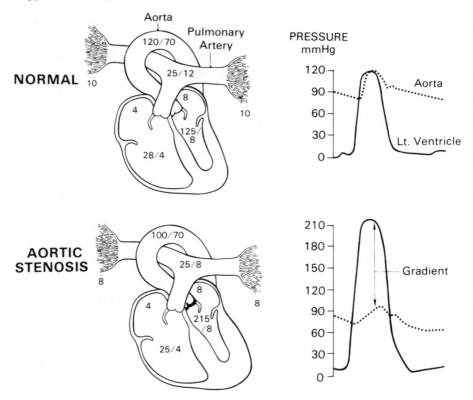

Figure 3-8. Left ventricular and aortic pressure gradients in a normal adult and in stenosis. Note in aortic stenosis the excessive left ventricular systolic pressure, the large systolic pressure gradient and the abnormally thickened left ventricle. ($\bar{X}$ = mean value.) (Adapted from an original painting by F. H. Netter, *Ciba Collection of Medical Illustrations,* vol. 5, Summit, N. J.: CIBA-Geigy Corp., 1955–1963).

of bronchial venous blood (from the lungs) and thebesian venous blood (from the myocardium), there is a small decrease in oxygen saturation in the left ventricle to about 95%. Normally, systemic arterial blood has the same oxygen content and saturation as left ventricular blood (Fig. 3-9).

In *ventricular septal defect,* a shunt of oxygenated blood occurs during systole from the left to the right ventricle through the septal defect, producing an abnormally high oxygen saturation in the right ventricle and frequently an abnormally high right ventricular pressure (Fig. 3-9, *right*). Eventually, if not repaired, the right ventricle may

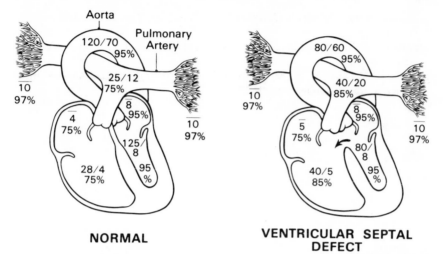

Figure 3-9. Intracardiac pressures and oxygen saturations in a normal adult and in ventricular septal defect. Because of the mixing of the two streams in ventricular septal defect, the left ventricular pressures are decreased and those on the right side of the heart are increased. Right ventricular and pulmonary arterial blood have a higher oxygen saturation. (Adapted from an original painting by F. H. Netter, *Ciba Collection of Medical Illustrations,* vol. 5, Summit, N. J.: CIBA-Geigy Corp., 1955–1963.)

become hypertrophied and the shunt may reverse to become a right to left shunt with cyanosis (a dusky or blue color of the skin) caused by a higher arterial blood concentration of reduced hemoglobin. The turbulence produced by blood flow through the septal defect during systole causes a systolic murmur.

REFERENCES

ARMOUR, J. A., AND W. C. RANDALL: Structural basis for cardiac function. *Am. J. Physiol.* 218:1517–1523, 1970.

BRECHER, G. A., AND P. M. GALLETTI: Functional anatomy of cardiac pumping. In *Handbook of Physiology,* Section 2: *Circulation,* vol. II, ed. by W. F. Hamilton and P. Dow, pp. 759–798. Washington, D.C.: American Physiological Society, 1963.

HURST, J. W. (Ed.): *The Heart, Arteries and Veins,* 3rd ed. New York: McGraw-Hill Book Co., 1974.

LEON, D. F., AND J. A. SHAVER (Eds.): *Physiologic Principles of Heart Sounds and Murmurs,* Monograph No. 46. Dallas: American Heart Association, 1974.

MOSKOVITZ, H. L., E. DONOSO, I. J. GELB, AND R. J. WILDER: *An Atlas of*

Hemodynamics of the Cardiovascular System. New York: Grune & Stratton, Inc., 1963.

RUSHMER, R. F.: *Cardiovascular Dynamics.* 4th ed. Philadelphia: W. B. Saunders Co., 1976.

SOKOLOW, M. AND M. B. McILROY: *Clinical Cardiology.* Los Altos, Calif.: Lange Medical Publications, 1977.

chapter 4

Pressure and Flow in the Arterial and Venous Systems

AORTIC PRESSURE AND FLOW

As indicated in the previous chapter (Fig. 3-6), during the first third of left ventricular emptying, about two thirds of the stroke volume is ejected into the aorta. Simultaneous aortic recordings with a pressure transducer and a sensitive flowmeter illustrate this rapid emptying as

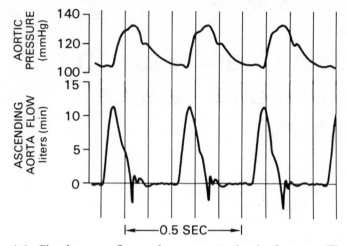

Figure 4-1. Simultaneous flow and pressure tracing in the aorta. There is a rapid ejection of blood from the left ventricle into the aorta followed by a rise in the aortic pressure. (From H. P. Peiper, *Rev. Sci. Instrum.* 29:965, 1958.)

a quick rise in aortic flow in early systole (Fig. 4-1). This rapid ejection is followed by a sharp fall in ejection rate; at the end of systole there is actually a small, transient reverse flow due to the influx of blood into the coronary arteries and to a lesser extent, to a slight regurgitation of blood back into the left ventricle through the aortic valve.

The pressure wave (Fig. 4-1, *upper*) is the shock impulse due to the sudden ejection of blood into the aorta; this wave is transmitted through the aortic blood column and aortic wall at a velocity of about 4 to 6 m/sec which is about 20 times greater than the mean velocity imparted to the blood itself (20 to 40 cm/sec). The pressure wave has, therefore, no direct relationship to flow and could occur fully as well if there were no flow at all. Because the transmission velocity of the pulse wave is increased when the arteries become less distensible, the speed of the wave has sometimes been used as a rough index of arterial distensibility.

Aortic Pressure Wave

Components

Because pressure is technically easier to record than flow and since the aorta stands midway between the heart and the circulatory beds of the tissues, the analysis of the aortic pressure wave can yield valuable information about both central and peripheral circulatory events.

The ascending or anacrotic limb of a typical aortic pressure wave (shown in Fig. 4-2) is the result of the forcible ejection of the left ventricular blood into the aorta with resultant distension of the aortic wall. After it reaches its peak, called the systolic pressure, the ventricular pressure declines to a level below the aortic (the catacrotic limb); at this point the aortic valve closes with a small rebound wave which marks the dicrotic notch and the end of ventricular systole. At a heart rate of 75 per minute, the cycle length is 0.8 sec or 800 msec, of which about three eighths or 0.3 sec is taken up by systole.

Diastole, which occupies the rest of the descending limb of the curve is characterized by a long, declining pressure wave during which the aortic wall recoils and propels blood distally to the tissues, the "diastolic runoff." Meanwhile the ventricle is relaxing and filling for the next stroke. Diastole occupies about five eighths of the cycle or 500

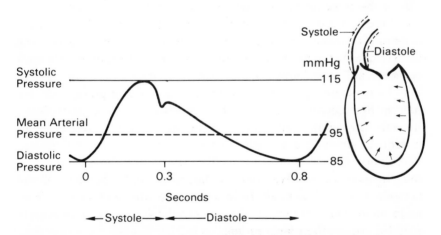

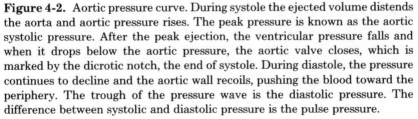

Figure 4-2. Aortic pressure curve. During systole the ejected volume distends the aorta and aortic pressure rises. The peak pressure is known as the aortic systolic pressure. After the peak ejection, the ventricular pressure falls and when it drops below the aortic pressure, the aortic valve closes, which is marked by the dicrotic notch, the end of systole. During diastole, the pressure continues to decline and the aortic wall recoils, pushing the blood toward the periphery. The trough of the pressure wave is the diastolic pressure. The difference between systolic and diastolic pressure is the pulse pressure.

msec; the lowest point of the pressure wave, which occurs at the end of isovolumic ventricular contraction, is called the diastolic pressure.

The difference between systolic and diastolic pressure is the pulse pressure. The mean aortic pressure is the average for the complete period, which is, in effect, the pressure-time integral for the entire cardiac cycle. The mean pressure can be determined electronically with a polygraph recorder or by determining the area under the curve (the pressure-time product) and dividing by the length of the cycle.

The true mean pressure in an artery is inevitably less than the arithmetic average of the systolic and diastolic pressures because the lower half of the curve has a greater area than the upper half. Under ordinary conditions and at normal heart rates, the mean arterial pressure can be roughly estimated as the diastolic pressure plus one third of the pulse pressure. Mean pressure values are essential for certain calculations, *e.g.*, in determining pressure gradients or peripheral resistance.

Transmission

Both the pressure values and the wave configurations are altered during transmission through the peripheral arterial tree (Fig. 4-3); with increasing distance from the heart, the dicrotic notch becomes less sharp (smoothed or filtered) and dicrotic waves appear. In the descending aorta and large arteries, the systolic pressures are higher and diastolic pressures are lower (with a resultant higher pulse pressure) than in the ascending aorta (Fig. 4-3); this is due at least partially, to the reflection of the pulse waves from the distal vascular bed and subsequent summation at those points.

It is important to note, however, that the mean pressure—the best single measure of effective driving pressure—is inevitably lower in the more distal arteries as might be expected at a point downstream from the pressure source; however, the pressure loss in the large arteries is small because of their large radius.

With further peripheral transmission and with progressive decrease in size of the arterial radii, the pulse waves are gradually dampened, particularly in the arterioles where the pressure reaches values of 40 to 60 mm Hg. The pulsatile characteristic of the pressure wave is ordinarily extinguished at the capillaries and veins; the venous pressure waves, which reappear in the large veins close to the heart, are similar

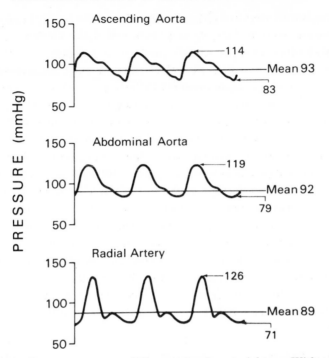

Figure 4-3. Pressure waves at different sites in arterial tree. With transmission of the pressure wave into the distal aorta and large arteries, the systolic pressure increases and the diastolic pressure decreases, with a resultant heightening of the pulse pressure. However, the mean arterial pressure declines steadily.

to the atrial waves (Chapter 3, Fig. 3-4) which are a backward transmission and reflect events of the right heart and not the left.

Determinants of Aortic Pressure

If the cardiac output (CO) is the ratio of the driving pressure ($\triangle P$) and the total peripheral resistance (TPR) and if we assume the vena cava pressure is approximately zero, then $\triangle P$ becomes mean aortic pressure (MAP) and we can (as stated in Chapter 2) formulate the generalization that: MAP = CO × TPR.

If the remaining factor is held constant, an increase or decrease in either cardiac output or total peripheral resistance will result in a corresponding increase or decrease in mean aortic pressure. Cardiac output may, in turn, be altered either by a change in heart rate or stroke volume so that changes in either of these factors may affect MAP depending on the net effect on cardiac output.

An analysis of the factors influencing arterial pressure (systolic, diastolic and mean) is important, partly because clinically, they may suggest the nature and site of hemodynamic disorders, and partly because in the cardiovascular system, arterial pressure is the prime "regulated variable." The latter refers to the fact that the major hemodynamic defense mechanisms which maintain circulatory function in case of stress or emergency (as will be discussed in Chapter 10) are triggered and controlled by the level of arterial pressure.

While mean pressure is a valuable measure, it is also possible to obtain useful information from the systolic and diastolic portions of the curve. Primary factors which produce and maintain the aortic pressure are listed in Figure 4-4. The relative importance of any single factor can only be determined if all other factors are held constant; since such conditions are usually not achievable in an intact circulation, the effects described below were determined mainly in circulatory models.

Systolic Pressure

The primary determinants of the systolic portion of the aortic pressure curve, *i.e.*, stroke volume, aortic distensibility and ejection

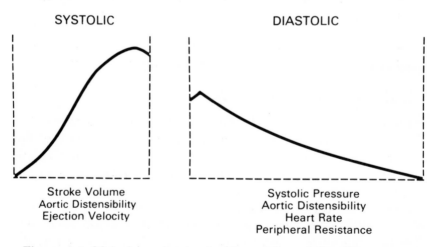

SYSTOLIC

Stroke Volume
Aortic Distensibility
Ejection Velocity

DIASTOLIC

Systolic Pressure
Aortic Distensibility
Heart Rate
Peripheral Resistance

Figure 4-4. Main determinants of aortic systolic and diastolic pressures.

velocity and their effects on aortic pressure are shown graphically in Figure 4-5.

Since about two thirds of the left ventricular stroke volume is temporarily retained in the aorta and large arteries after ventricular ejection, the resultant pressure changes in the aorta have been estimated in Figure 4-5 on the basis of aortic distensibility (volume-pressure) relationships discussed in Chapter 1. Using this approach, certain generalizations are possible, *e.g.*, an increase in stroke volume will cause an increase in aortic pressure and also an increase in the area under the systolic portion of the aortic pressure curve (Fig. 4-5

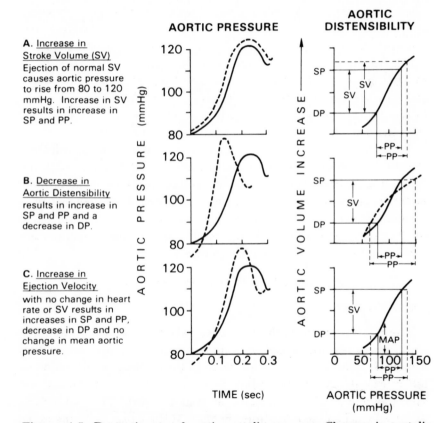

Figure 4-5. Determinants of aortic systolic pressure. Changes in systolic pressure (SP), diastolic pressure (DP) and pulse pressure (PP) with alterations in stroke volume (SV), aortic distensibility and ejection velocity. Figures are diagrammatic and indicate general tendencies if other factors are held constant.

upper). However, a change in aortic distensibility as seen, *e.g.*, with advancing age (Chapter 1, Fig. 1-8) will result in a higher systolic pressure and a lesser diastolic pressure, *i.e.*, a greater pulse pressure, at equivalent aortic volumes (Fig. 4-5 *middle*). More rapid ejection (Fig. 4-5 *lower*) will similarly cause greater pulse pressures because of inadequate time for the aortic wall to distend in response to the ejected volume.

Diastolic Pressure

The determinants of diastolic pressure are shown in Figure 4-6. With other factors held constant, increase in systolic pressure, produced, *e.g.*, by increased stroke volume, will elevate the entire pressure curve and increase diastolic pressure (Fig. 4-6*A*). With decreased aortic distensibility, the lack of recoil will not sustain the diastolic pressure, which will then fall off more rapidly (Fig. 4-6*B*). An increased heart rate will interrupt the diastolic decline at a higher point on the curve and raise the diastolic pressure (Fig. 4-6*C*); if cardiac output is thereby increased, the systolic pressure will also increase but probably less than the diastolic so that there is a fall in pulse pressure.

An increased peripheral resistance, as previously noted, will raise the mean arterial pressure and also systolic and diastolic pressure. Again it must be emphasized that in the intact organism, two or more factors may coexist and compensatory reflex responses may be superimposed. However, changes in the systolic and diastolic pressures and in the wave configuration may provide useful clues to important central and peripheral circulatory changes.

ARTERIAL BLOOD PRESSURE

Pulse Pressure

The pulse pressure is the difference between the systolic and diastolic pressures and would, of course, not exist in a constant flow system. It is due to the force imparted to the arterial blood column by left ventricular contraction which produces a pressure increment over and above the existing diastolic arterial pressure. The pulse wave excursions, when recorded from the body surface (*e.g.*, over the radial artery at the wrist) are damped versions of the arterial pressure wave. The area of the wave will be roughly proportional to the ventricular stroke volume and the character of the wave, *e.g.*, the upstroke, will

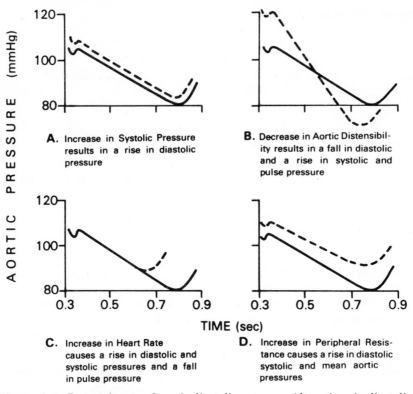

Figure 4-6. Determinants of aortic diastolic pressure. Alterations in diastolic pressure resulting from changes in systolic pressure, aortic distensibility, heart rate and peripheral resistance. Figures are diagrammatic indicating general tendencies if other factors are held constant.

generally reflect aortic distensibility and ejection velocity, as previously described.

Although more precise information about the heart can be obtained from the ECG, heart sounds and blood pressure, palpation of the pulse at the carotid or radial artery can give general indications of: (a) *Rate and rhythm of the heart*—extra systoles may be detected if the ejection is forceful enough to transmit the impulse to the periphery; (b) *Pulse pressure*—often will be increased in advanced arteriosclerosis or aortic regurgitation; it will be decreased in deep shock in which the rapid, "thready" pulse is characteristic; (c) *Approximate level of arterial pressure*—may be gauged by the tension required to obliterate the pulse entirely with one finger while palpating with an adjacent finger.

Normal Values

In the foregoing section, emphasis has been placed on the components of arterial pressure and the central and peripheral hemodynamic factors which may affect arterial pressure in an acute situation. There are other factors which affect arterial pressure on a long term basis. Some individuals, more responsive to stress, may show rather wide variations in arterial blood pressure; in such instances repeated daily measurements after a brief rest period will help to determine the true normal value for that individual.

Age is an important factor; with advancing years there is a progressive tendency toward increase in both systolic and diastolic pressures (Fig. 4-7). Indications of abnormal values should be checked by repeated determinations. The problem of hypertension is discussed in Chapter 15.

VENOUS SYSTEM: PRESSURE-VOLUME-FLOW RELATIONS

As previously mentioned (Chapter 1) the venous system has about five to six times greater distensibility and about two to three times greater capacity than the arterial system. Thus its capacitance, *i.e.,* the unit volume it will accommodate per unit pressure (dV/dP), is about 15 times greater than that of the arterial tree. Consequently,

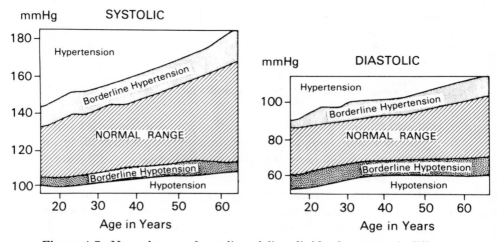

Figure 4-7. Normal range of systolic and diastolic blood pressures in different age groups. (From R. F. Rushmer, *Cardiovascular Dynamics,* 4th ed. Philadelphia: W.B. Saunders Co., 1976.)

when blood or plasma is infused into the vascular system, these fluids, since they seek pressure equilibrium, tend rather rapidly to distribute themselves in the venous and arterial system in the same ratio, *i.e.*, about 15:1. Similarly in case of hemorrhage, the decrease in vascular volume is predominantly on the venous side. This can be demonstrated either *in vivo* or in an artificial system containing tubes of similar distensibilities and capacities (Fig. 4-8).

VENOUS RETURN TO THE HEART

The factors influencing venous return may be classified into two general divisions, *i.e.*, primary and secondary. The primary and by far the dominant factor is the pressure transmitted from the left ventricle through the arteries and veins to the right atrium. Secondary factors are (a) the skeletal muscle pump, (b) the respiratory pump, (c) the venous valves, (d) the "suction" effect of ventricular contraction and relaxation on the atria and (e) venomotor tone, *i.e.*, the state of contraction or relaxation of the smooth muscle of the veins.

Primary Factor Influencing Venous Return

The dominant force which drives blood back to the heart has been called the systemic filling pressure (P_{SF}), *i.e.*, the "mean circulatory

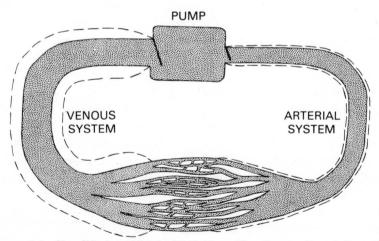

Figure 4-8. Simplified artificial circulation. The "venous" and "arterial" tubes have capacitance ratios of 15 to 1. Upon overfilling the system, the additional fluid distributes itself in about the same ratio.

pressure" of the systemic circuit. The P_{SF} represents the hemodynamic gradient for the entire systemic circulation, from the root of the aorta to the right atrium; its value is about 7 mm Hg in man. The net driving pressure returning blood to the heart can then be visualized as the difference between the P_{SF} and right atrial pressure. The P_{SF} and its role in venous return is discussed further in Chapter 7.

Secondary Factors Influencing Venous Return

Skeletal Muscle Pump

In certain situations, e.g., in adjustment to the erect posture, skeletal muscles play a significant role. Immediately upon standing, blood gravitates toward the veins of the lower extremity; the venous valves temporarily prevent this retrograde flow but the veins fill rapidly from below. Within a few seconds they are engorged and the pressures in the foot and ankle veins increase to reflect the increased height of the hydrostatic blood column. Shortly thereafter the skeletal muscles of the lower extremity begin rather rhythmical cycles of reflex contraction and relaxation which are responsible for the unconscious swaying action of the body during quiet standing; this materially assists the venous return and helps to redress the pooling effect of gravity. Lifting of one foot off the ground will increase the venous pressure in that foot but swinging of the leg will accelerate venous return and reduce local venous pressure; upon quiet standing, the venous pressure will again rise (Fig. 4-9A). Upon walking, skeletal muscle action will milk the blood centralward and lower the volume and pressure in the dependent veins; however, with cessation of movement, the venous pressure will again rise (Fig. 4-9B) at a rate which depends on the rate of arteriolar inflow to the leg. At a comfortable external temperature (skin temperature of 25°C) the inflow rate is relatively low and the rate of rise of venous pressure is a shallow one (Fig. 4-9B); however, if the outside temperature is higher and the skin temperature rises, the arterioles will dilate, the inflow rate will rise, venous flow will increase and the venous pressure rise will be steeper (dashed line).

In order for the lower extremity muscles to serve as an effective pump, it is necessary for the feet to anchor the body so that skeletal muscles may have a counterweight against which to contract. The importance of this auxiliary pump is underscored by the fact that if the body is suspended in an upright position so that the feet dangle and cannot reach the ground, this unconscious milking action of lower

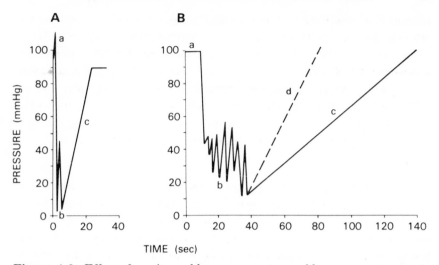

A **B**

PRESSURE (mmHg)

TIME (sec)

Figure 4-9. Effect of gravity and leg movement on ankle venous pressure. *A.* Shows venous pressure when heel is off ground (*a*), when leg swings free (*b*) and with heel on ground (*c*). *B.* Ankle venous pressure at quiet standing (*a*), with walking (*b*) and gradual increase again with quiet standing (*c*), or with an increased flow rate e.g. at higher temperatures (*d*), (Adapted from A. A. Pollack and E. H. Wood, *J. Appl. Physiol.* 1:649, 1948–1949; and from J. P. Henry and O. Gauer, *J. Clin. Invest.* 29:855, 1950.)

extremity muscles is largely prevented; in this situation most individuals suffer marked reduction of venous return and cardiac output. A 30- to 60-minute suspension in this fashion will produce fainting and a longer exposure may be life-threatening. The ancient practice of execution by crucifixion was largely based on the resultant circulatory stress from upright suspension.

On the other hand, massive and widespread skeletal muscle contraction may produce excessive venous return and temporarily an increased cardiac output.

Respiratory Pump

This refers to the assistance given to venous return by the mechanical movements of respiration. The intrathoracic pressure is usually slightly subatmospheric and varies during quiet breathing from about −2 to −4 mm Hg during expiration to about −5 to −7 mm Hg during inspiration. As the intrathoracic pressure falls, the intraabdominal pressure rises due to the descent of the diaphragm. The changes in pressure gradient facilitate venous return from outside the thorax during inspiration and diminish it during expiration. In this process, during inspiration, the venous return to the right heart increases but due to the simultaneously increased volume and capacitance of the pulmonary arterial bed, the return of blood to the left heart decreases.

These tendencies are exaggerated with heightening of the respiratory movements and the consequent increases in respiratory pressure increments; however, the effect is limited because of the likelihood of venous collapse at the point of entrance of the veins into the thorax if intravenous pressure becomes negative at that level (Chapter 7).

Venous Valves

Venous valves are very thin, transparent, cusplike structures in the veins of the extremities which insure unidirectional flow. The venous valves are a very significant aid to venous return and when, as may occur particularly in the lower extremity, they are subjected to prolonged increases in venous pressures incident to pregnancy or prolonged standing, they may become incompetent; this, in turn, may lead to varicosities and other local circulatory disturbances because of deficient venous drainage.

"Suction" Effect of Ventricular Contraction and Relaxation on the Atria

While the P_{SF} is the main force driving blood toward the heart, the ventricles also contribute to venous return through a negative or suction effect exerted in the opposite direction. During ventricular systole, when the AV valves are closed, the AV junction is drawn downward by the ventricles, enlarging the atria, thereby lowering its relative internal pressure and thus increasing flow from the vena cavae and pulmonary veins. Current evidence further indicates that during diastole, the ventricles also exert a negative pressure by virtue of the "diastolic recoil" of their walls.

Venomotor Tone

The state of contraction of the venous smooth muscle is a significant factor in venous return because a small increase in tone or contractile state, *e.g.*, through venoconstriction, can shift a large amount of blood toward the heart. In certain stresses, *e.g.*, hemorrhage, reflex venoconstriction is a very important compensatory response (Chapters 10 and 13).

VENOUS PRESSURE

Measurement

Venous pressures, either peripheral or central, may be determined by intravascular catheterization. Because the venous pressures are relatively low, either water manometers or more sensitive pressure transducers (discussed below) are often employed. As previously mentioned, the pulsatile arterial pressure is ordinarily damped out and becomes non-pulsatile at the capillary level. Pressures in the venules and larger peripheral veins are also non-pulsatile; mean values range from 10 to 15 mm Hg in small venules, 4 to 8 mm Hg in peripheral veins and from −2 to +2 mm Hg in the vena cavae. Within the vena cavae, pulsations again appear and resemble the pressure wave pattern seen in the right atrium (Fig. 3-4, Chapter 3).

Gravity Effect on Venous Pressure

Since the circulatory system is closed and in this sense resembles a U tube or siphon, it should be pointed out that the driving pressure, in contrast to the transmural pressure, is not influenced by gravity but depends only on the difference between the inlet and outlet pressures, *i.e.*, those at the root of the aorta and the vena caval entrance to the heart.

The effective driving pressure at any point propelling blood toward the heart will, therefore, be the ambient pressure minus the gravity pressure; all intravascular pressures must be so "corrected" by adding or subtracting the vertical height of the fluid column, but the correction is particularly important in the case of the venous pressure. Upon quiet standing, the foot vein in a normal adult, being about 120 cm below the heart, will, therefore, have an additional pressure of 120 cm of H_2O (*i.e.*, about 88 mm Hg) (Fig. 4-10).

Thus if the ambient pressure in a foot vein at rest is 102 mm Hg, the effective driving pressure will be 14 mm Hg. (However, as previously mentioned, during movement such as walking, skeletal muscle action will break up the vertical gravity column and temporarily reduce the pressure.) The large hydrostatic pressure in the dependent vessels might be expected to increase transmural pressure, increase capillary transudation and produce edema (Chapter 8); however, this gravity

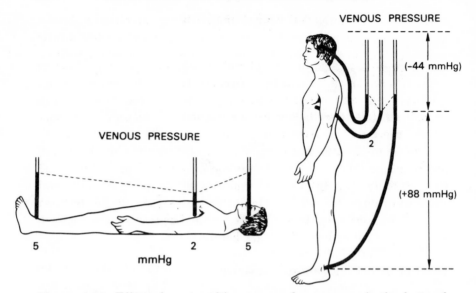

Figure 4-10. Effect of erect position on vascular pressures in the foot and head. Pressures taken in the lower part of the body should be corrected by subtracting the pressure equivalent of the vertical distance below the heart. (From A. C. Burton, *Physiology and Biophysics of the Circulation*, 2nd ed. Chicago: Year Book Medical Publishers Inc., 1972.)

effect is largely offset by the extravascular gravity effect on interstitial tissue fluid in the leg and also by the skeletal muscle pump and venous valve action.

Similarly, pressures above the heart must be corrected by adding the appropriate hydrostatic pressure. However, in the cranium, changes in transmural pressure as well as in cerebral blood flow are minimized during gravity changes by (a) the close equilibrium between the cerebral veins and the cerebrospinal fluid (Chapter 11), (b) the fact that both systems are confined within a relatively rigid chamber and (c) the attachment of the dural sinuses which prevents their collapse in case they are subjected to negative transmural pressures.

Disturbances of Venous Pressure and Flow

In certain pathological situations, venous flow will be diminished through compression of abdominal or thoracic veins, *e.g.*, by pregnancy or tumors. Unusual respiratory efforts such as coughing, straining at stool, blowing of a musical instrument or strong expiration against a fixed resistance can induce large transitory increases in intrathoracic pressure; this, in turn, can markedly reduce venous return, cardiac output and arterial pressure (see Valsalva Test, Chapter 13).

BLOOD FLOW MEASUREMENT: METHODS

Because the interpretation of blood flow and blood pressure data is closely linked with how the data were obtained, a brief review will be made of the more common methods in current use. Flow methods applicable to cardiac output, *i.e.*, central blood flow, will be discussed in Chapter 7; following is a brief description of the principles involved in sensing peripheral flow.

Electromagnetic Flowmeter. This invasive method is widely used in experimental studies to determine pulsatile flow in individual arteries (Fig. 4-11). A collar or probe which has two small electrodes positioned on opposite sides of the artery is placed around the blood vessel. Two small magnets, also incorporated into the probe, produce a constant magnetic field across the blood vessel; if a conductor such as blood moves through this field, the electric potential developed at the electrodes is proportional to the velocity of the stream. Knowing the cross-sectional area of the vessel, the volume flow per minute can be

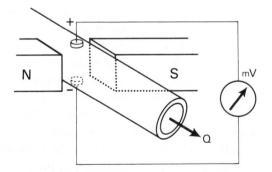

Figure 4-11. Principle of the electromagnetic flowmeter. When a conducting fluid containing ions flows through a magnetic field, an electromagnetic force will be generated perpendicular to the field and proportional to the velocity of the fluid. (From T. C. Ruch and H. D. Patton, *Physiology and Biophysics.* Philadelphia: W. B. Saunders Co., 1974.)

calculated. This is an excellent method for accurate flow measurement in an isolated vessel and is particularly applicable to animal studies.

Ultrasonic Flowmeter. There has been increasing interest in the use of ultrasound for a variety of biological measurements including the detection of arterial and venous flow. High frequency sound waves are directed across the vessel and transmitted both downstream and upstream. There is a shift in frequency of the sound, depending on the velocity of flow, which is called the Doppler effect. By detecting the relative velocities of these sound transmissions, the volume flow in the blood vessel can be estimated knowing the cross-sectional area of the vessel. One advantage of the ultrasonic method is that the detector can be positioned on the surface of the body so that blood flow may be determined in a non-invasive manner.

Impedance Flowmeter. If band electrodes are placed about a limb, *e.g.*, the calf, and the electrodes excited by a high frequency (100 kHz) sinusoidal current, the observed voltage and impedance changes are dependent on the velocity of blood flow. From the impedance wave forms, the volume flow through the limb may be calculated. The low amplitude, high frequency current has no injurious effect on the tissues; the impedance method is also adaptable for non-invasive determination of cardiac output (see Chapter 7, Impedance Cardiography).

Venous Occlusion Plethysmography. This method is particularly suitable for blood flow determination in an intact limb (Fig. 4-12). By enclosing the extremity in an airtight container and sealing the skin junction, sudden temporary occlusion of the venous return with an occlusion cuff will permit, by means of a sensitive recorder, the registration of the volume change of the limb per unit of time. Since a temporary venous occlusion will not affect arterial flow, this limb volume change will, for the first 6 to 8 seconds, faithfully record the arterial inflow to the limb. The determination can be repeated after relatively short intervals. By means of a temporary arterial tourniquet at the wrist or ankle, the hand or foot blood flow, which is primarily skin flow, can be excluded; this will permit flow measurements on the forearm or calf alone, which consist primarily of skeletal muscle tissue. This is a convenient and useful non-invasive method in which flows to different tissues of a limb can be determined, for example, in patients with peripheral vascular disease.

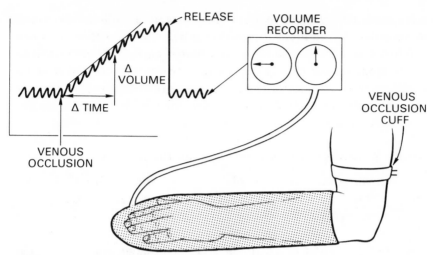

Figure 4-12. Venous occlusion plethysmograph. When the cuff is rapidly inflated to 50 mm Hg, venous outflow is prevented and for the next few seconds, the volume increase in the plethysmograph will reflect the arterial inflow. The initial slope of increased volume per unit time on the calibrated volume recorder will indicate the blood flow to the forearm in milliliters per minute.

BLOOD PRESSURE MEASUREMENT: METHODS

In the preceding chapters, calculations of resistance have usually been based on pressure-flow relations as they exist in a constant flow circuit. However, to assess more precisely the resistance to pulsatile flow in the arterial system, it must be treated as dynamic resistance, *i.e.*, as impedance to flow. Vascular impedance, if determined as the ratio of mean pressure to mean flow at one point such as the root of the aorta, provides an impedance value at only one frequency, *i.e.*, zero, which is the resistance. However, the pressure and flow velocities vary and their relationship will also vary depending not only on fluid characteristics such as viscosity and on vessel wall composition and geometry, but also with the frequency, *i.e.*, heart rate. Thus, a more precise determination of hindrance to flow would necessitate the analysis of pressure to flow characteristics at the multiple frequencies which exist in the arterial system.

This complex problem has been studied by means of mathematical analysis of the pressure and flow waves; assuming periodic, sinusoidal wave motion, harmonic analysis has been used to generate models which simulate the arterial system and help to understand such flow and pressure relations. Although adequate *in vivo* data in the circulatory system are scarce, this approach has provided some estimates of aortic resistance to left ventricular emptying (afterload) and the impedance effects of such afterloads on myocardial performance in congestive heart failure.

Direct Methods of Measuring Arterial Blood Pressure

This involves the placement of a needle or catheter directly into the artery. Pressure and flow studies in a pulsatile system (as described in the previous section) have helped to clarify the requirements for such direct arterial pressure recording. In order to adequately register pressure fluctuations at a given heart rate, a manometer system must have several characteristics, including adequate band width, which is the ability to faithfully reproduce at least the first five harmonics; the system must, therefore, be able to respond to frequencies about five times that of the heart rate.

The strain gauge pressure transducer, which is commonly employed for such arterial pressure sensing, consists of a stiff diaphragm to which are bonded several strain gauges capable of responding rapidly to the transient pressure changes. The hydraulic system which couples the transducer to the artery by means of a catheter is an important element; to retain maximum sensitivity, it should be of maximum bore and of minimum length in order to avoid excessive damping of the pressure wave.

The direct method provides the most accurate pressure data; however, it is invasive and, since it involves the placement of a catheter in the vessel, requires that the procedure be performed under sterile conditions.

Indirect Blood Pressure Methods

These are most commonly used because of their practicability and ease of repetition. The method depends either (a) on the production of Korotkoff sounds, which are mainly the result of turbulence in the stream, or (b) on the appearance and disappearance of the pulse upon palpation (Fig. 4-13).

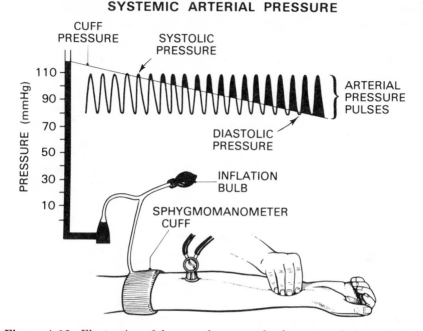

Figure 4-13. Illustration of the auscultatory and palpatory techniques for the indirect method of measuring arterial blood pressure. The appearance and disappearance of the auscultatory sounds are illustrated. (From E. E. Selkurt, *Physiology*, 4th ed. Boston: Little, Brown and Co., 1976.)

The instrument used is a sphygmomanometer that consists of an inelastic cuff which encloses a rubber bag. Inflation of the cuff to a level above systolic pressure will occlude all blood flow to and from the arm; gradual reduction of the cuff pressure will permit a return of arterial flow as detected by the appearance of an audible tapping sound at the brachial artery below the cuff, which marks the systolic pressure. Progressive decrease of the pressure will produce characteristic sound fluctuations (Fig. 4-14) and finally muffling and disappearance of the sound which marks diastolic pressure; whether muffling or disappearance is the more valid measure is not certain. Usually both are recorded so the blood pressure would read, *e.g.*, 124/80/74. In some instances, during the lowering of cuff pressure, the sounds may temporarily disappear and then reappear, a possible source of error in the determination (auscultatory gap, Fig. 4-14). To avoid errors in reading,

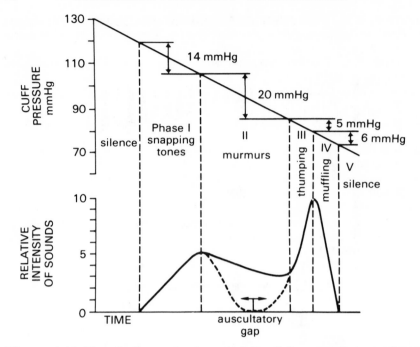

Figure 4-14. Korotkoff sounds characteristic of the auscultatory phases during measurement of blood pressure in the human. (Reproduced with permission from L. A. Geddes, *The Direct and Indirect Measurement of Blood Pressure*. Chicago: Year Book Medical Publishers Inc., 1970.)

the cuff must be of sufficient width in order to fully transmit the applied pressure to the arteries of the limb. It is generally agreed that the cuff must be at least 20% wider than the diameter of the limb.

Although the indirect method does not provide a continuous recording and is not as accurate as the direct, it is rapid and convenient and if carefully performed serves adequately in most clinical circumstances.

REFERENCES

ALEXANDER, R. S.: The peripheral venous system. In *Handbook of Physiology*, Section 2: *Circulation*, vol. II, ed. by W. F. Hamilton and P. Dow, p. 1075. Washington, D.C.: American Physiological Society, 1963.

FOLKOW, B., AND E. NEIL: *Circulation*. London: Oxford Medical Press, 1971.

FRY, D. L.: Flow detection techniques. In *Methods in Medical Research*, ed. by R. F. Rushmer. Chicago: Year Book Medical Publishers, Inc., 1966.

GAUER, O.: Properties of veins in vivo. *Physiol. Rev.* 42:283, 1962.

GEDDES, L. A.: *Direct and Indirect Measurement of Blood Pressure*. Chicago: Year Book Medical Publishers, Inc., 1970.

GUYTON, A. C., C. E. JONES, AND T. E. COLEMAN: *Circulatory Physiology: Cardiac Output and Its Regulation*, 2nd ed., Philadelphia: W. B. Saunders Co., 1973.

GUYTON, A. C.: *Textbook of Medical Physiology*, 5th ed. Philadelphia: W. B. Saunders Co., 1976.

MILNOR, W. R.: Arterial impedance as ventricular afterload. *Circ. Res.* 36:565, 1975.

PATEL, D. J., R. N. VAISHNAV, B. S. GOW, AND P. A. KOT: Hemodynamics. *Annu. Rev. Physiol.* 36:125–154, 1974.

ROACH, M. R.: Biophysical analyses of blood vessel walls and blood flow. *Annu. Rev. Physiol.* 39:51–72, 1977.

STRANDNESS, D. E., AND D. S. SUMNER: *Hemodynamics for Surgeons*. New York: Grune & Stratton Inc., 1975.

SPENCER, M. P., AND A. B. DENISON: Pulsatile blood flow in vascular system. In *Handbook of Physiology*, Section 2: *Circulation*, vol. II, ed. by W. F. Hamilton and P. Dow, p. 839. Washington, D.C.: American Physiological Society, 1963.

chapter 5

Electrical Properties of the Heart

SPREAD OF THE CARDIAC IMPULSE

As was discussed in Chapter 3, the heart normally beats in an orderly sequence so that atrial systole is followed by ventricular systole. This sequential coordination is brought about by a specialized cardiac conduction system which consists of the sinoatrial (SA) node, atrial bundles, the atrioventricular (AV) node, the bundle of His with its right and left branches and the Purkinje network. The SA node, the AV node, and the remaining specialized conduction tissue can all discharge spontaneously, *i.e.*, can initiate action potentials and serve as "pacemakers." However, the SA node ordinarily has the fastest discharge rate and as a consequence, is the normal cardiac pacesetter or pacemaker. The location of the different elements of this system are shown in Figure 5-1 (*left*).

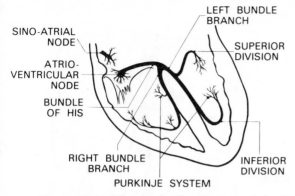

SITE	EXCITATION TIME (msec)
SA NODE	0
AV NODE	66
BUNDLE OF HIS	130
ANT SURFACE RT VENT	190
APICAL SURFACE	220
POSTERIOR LEFT VENT	260

Figure 5-1. The conduction system of the heart. *Left*, the action potential normally originates at the sinoatrial (SA) node, travels over the atria to the atrioventricular (AV) node and then through the bundle of His, the bundle branches and the Purkinje system to the ventricular muscle. *Right*, the time of arrival of the action potential at different parts of the heart. (Reproduced with permission from M. J. Goldman, *Principles of Clinical Electrocardiography*, 10th ed., 1978. Copyright 1978 by Lange Medical Publications, Los Altos, Calif.)

The transmission velocity in the SA node is about 0.05 m/sec and in the atrial muscle, bundle of His and ventricular muscle 0.8 to 1.0 m/sec. The conduction velocity in the AV node is 0.03 to 0.05 m/sec; however, in the Purkinje tissue it is 5 m/sec, *i.e.*, about 100 times greater than in the nodal systems. The impulse transmission times to the various regions are shown in Figure 5-1 (*right*).

THE ACTION POTENTIAL AT DIFFERENT SITES

As with other living cells, the action potential (AP) in the myocardial cell is generated by a series of changes in membrane conductance; the conductance changes, in turn, are initiated by a fall in the resting potential toward the threshold potential. There are, however, important differences in the APs of various cardiac tissues. The characteristic AP of ventricular muscle (non-pacemaker tissue) shows a rapid initial depolarization from about −90 mV to about +10 mV (phase 0), a quick partial repolarization and then a "plateau" voltage near zero (phase 2) which is maintained for several hundred milliseconds. This is followed by a rapid repolarization (phase 3) (Fig. 5-2*D*).

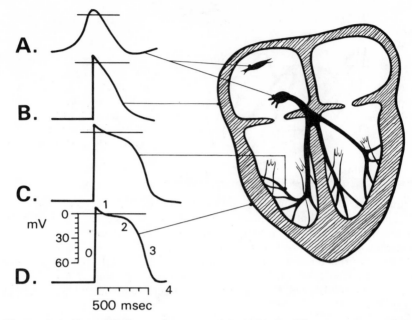

Figure 5-2. Intracellular action potentials (AP) in different regions of the heart. The pacemaker type of potential (sinoatrial or atrioventricular node) is shown in *A*, the atrial AP in *B*, the Purkinje fiber potential in *C* and ventricular cell AP in *D*. Zero voltage shown by *horizontal lines*. Note the depolarization potential and lack of plateau in the pacemaker tissue (*A*). The different phases of the AP are sometimes identified by numbers as shown in *D*. (From T. C. Ruch, H. D. Patton, and A. M. Scher (Eds.), *Physiology and Biophysics.* Philadelphia: W.B. Saunders Co., 1974.)

PACEMAKER POTENTIALS

The most important characteristic of the pacemaker AP is a slow membrane depolarization during diastole which precedes the initiation of the action potential (Fig. 5-3). This depolarization potential between APs—called the "pacemaker potential"—has an important influence on heart rate. Note in Figure 5-4 the spontaneous diastolic depolarization between *a* and *b* in pacemaker cell (*A*) but not in ventricular muscle cell (*B*).

The heart rate may slow through (a) decrease in the slope of diastolic depolarization (b) a rise in the threshold potential (TP-1 to TP-2 in Fig. 5-3) or (c) an increase in the magnitude of the resting potential

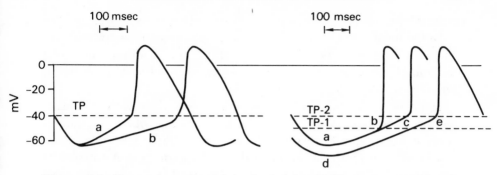

Figure 5-3. Pacemaker potentials in sinoatrial node. Illustrating the effect of diastolic depolarization slopes and potentials on heart rate. The action potential is initiated when the depolarization potential reaches threshold potential (TP). *Left*, slowing of rate of depolarization from *a* to *b* increases the time required to reach TP and lessens heart rate. *Right*, increase of level of TP from 1 to 2 or increased magnitude of resting potential from *a* to *d* also slows the discharge rate and, therefore, the heart rate. (From B. F. Hoffman and P. F. Cranefield, *Electrophysiology of the Heart.* New York: McGraw-Hill Book Co., 1960. Used with permission of McGraw-Hill Book Co.)

(*a* to *d*, Fig. 5-3, *right*). All these factors increase the length of time it takes the pacemaker potential to reach threshold; this results in a decreased rate of AP discharge and thus a decrease in heart rate. Conversely, opposite changes will increase the heart rate.

The heart rate may also be altered by a shift in pacemaker site. Inactivation of the normal pacemaker, *e.g.*, in sinus node disorders or AV block, will permit latent pacemakers such as Purkinje fibers or the ventricular muscle near pacemaker sites to become "ectopic foci" and assume pacemaker function by default. Such latent pacemakers have lower resting membrane potentials and smaller action potentials and drive the heart at a lower frequency than the normal pacemaker.

ELECTRICAL AND IONIC EVENTS OF CONTRACTION

The resting polarized membrane is relatively permeable to K^+; when depolarized by an outward flow of current, Na^+ conductance increases sharply and a net inward flux of Na^+ occurs down its concentration gradient; Na^+ ions enter the cell faster than the K^+ ions can leave, thus causing the membrane potential to overshoot above zero to levels of +10 or +20 mV. The Na^+ permeability now falls quickly and K^+

permeability rises; in many excitable tissues (*e.g.*, nerve fiber) this rise in K^+ permeability restores the resting potential within a few milliseconds but in cardiac tissue it takes several hundred milliseconds. The relation of these ionic events to the pacemaker potential is shown in Figure 5-4.

At present it is thought that pacemaker cells possess their characteristics because of (a) a relatively high resting diastolic Na^+ conductance, and (b) a slow decline in K^+ conductance during diastole.

A significant ionic change in cardiac cells during the AP (which is not shown in Fig. 5-4) is a slow inward current of Ca^{++} ions into the cell during the plateau period. The slowness of the repolarization of the cardiac cell and the resultant prolongation of the action potential is due to the slow inward Ca^{++} current which opposes the repolarizing

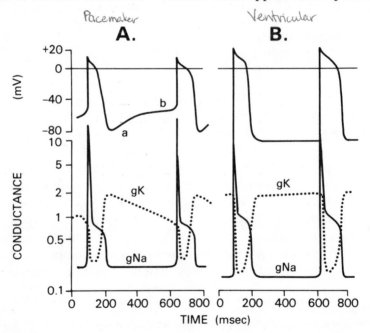

Figure 5-4. Relationship between electrical and ionic events during action potential (AP) in pacemaker cells (*A*) and ventricular cells (*B*). There is a sharp increase in sodium conductance (gNa) and a decrease in potassium conductance (gK) during the spike of the AP in rabbit heart and a reversal of these tendencies shortly thereafter. In the nodal tissue (*A*) during diastole there is a higher resting gNa and a tendency toward decline of gK. (From W. Trautwein, *Pharmacol. Rev.* 15:277, 1963.)

effect of the extrusion of Na^+ from the cell. The inward Ca^{++} migration also makes the Ca^{++} ions more available for excitation and contraction coupling—an essential part of the contraction process which is further described in Chapter 6.

ELECTRICAL AND MECHANICAL EVENTS OF CONTRACTION

A cell is refractory, *i.e.*, is unable to respond to a stimulus, if the stimulus arrives during depolarization or the initial phase of repolarization, *i.e.*, if the voltage of the cell has not become sufficiently negative to initiate the next AP. When the intracellular voltage is greater than about −50 mV, no matter how strong the stimulus there will be no inward Na^+ current and no new AP so that the cell is totally unexcitable. This is called the absolute refractory period (Fig. 5-5). Because the duration of this prolonged refractoriness is of the same order of

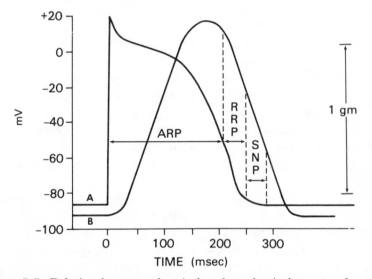

Figure 5-5. Relation between electrical and mechanical events of cardiac contraction showing the transmembrane action potential (AP) (*A*) in isolated papillary muscle and the subsequent isometric contraction curve (*B*). There is a considerable delay between the spike of the AP and the peak of the contraction. The graph also shows the refractoriness of the muscle to a subsequent stimulation. ARP, absolute refractory period; RRP, relative refractory period; and SNP, supernormal period. (Adapted from J. M. Marshall, Vertebrate smooth muscle. In *Medical Physiology*, 13th ed., ed. by V. B. Mountcastle. St. Louis: C.V. Mosby Co., 1974.)

magnitude as the duration of contraction, the heart cannot be tetanized. As the voltage of the cell becomes more negative (during the latter part of repolarization) it requires a stronger than normal stimulus to evoke a response; this is the "relative refractory period" (RRP). Immediately following the RRP there is—particularly in the Purkinje fiber—a supernormal phase of increased excitability. The refractory period varies in different parts of the heart, being shortest in the atrium and longest in the Purkinje system and AV node.

EXTRINSIC INFLUENCES ON THE HEART

The heart has innate automaticity and rhythmicity which is independent of neural influences; however, extrinsic factors—neural, thermal, metabolic and ionic—can and do significantly influence cardiac function.

Neural Effects

Vagal stimulation or acetylcholine (ACh) will (a) slow the heart, (b) decrease the strength of atrial contraction, and (c) cause a marked reduction in conduction velocity through the AV node. The rate effect is due to an increase in membrane permeability to K^+ which accelerates the repolarization phase of the AP, hyperpolarizes the membrane and decreases the slope of diastolic depolarization. Strong vagal stimulation will arrest the heart; however, even with continued stimulation the normal heart will, after a short interval, again resume beating (vagal escape).

Sympathetic stimulation or administration of norepinephrine or epinephrine will (a) increase the rate and force of cardiac contraction, (b) increase the conduction velocity through the AV node, atria and ventricles, and (c) increase the tendency of Purkinje fibers to exhibit pacemaker activity (Fig. 5-6). The rate effect is due to an increased rate (or slope) of membrane depolarization in the SA node. The myocardial action of catecholamines is due, in part at least, to stimulation of the intracellular enzyme, adenyl cyclase; the resultant reactions involve increased concentration of 3'5 AMP in the myocardial cell and ultimately the Ca^{++} accumulation rate of the reticulum is enhanced. Systole is thereby shortened and the contraction strengthened.

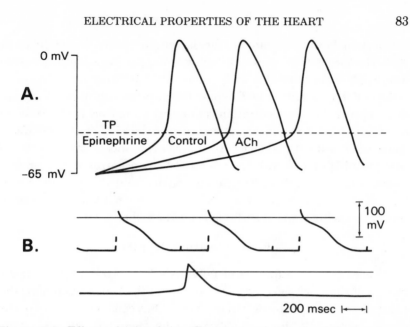

Figure 5-6. Effects of epinephrine (E) or sympathetic stimulation, and acetylcholine (ACh) or vagal stimulation on heart rate (A) and Purkinje fiber
action potentials (AP) (B). E increases and ACh decreases the slope of diastolic
depolarization (A). E converts Purkinje fiber APs (B, *upper strip*) to pacemaker
type (B, *lower strip*). (From E. E. Selkurt, *Physiology*, 4th ed. Boston: Little,
Brown & Co., 1976.)

Temperature

Warming the SA node increases its spontaneous activity and its
slope of diastolic depolarization, thereby speeding heart rate. There is
approximately a 10 beat/min rate increase per 1°C elevation of temperature. Cooling has the reverse effect and severe cooling may arrest
the heart.

Inorganic Ions

As Ringer showed many years ago, a proper extracellular concentration and balance of ions are essential for normal cardiac functioning.
As the plasma K^+ level rises (*e.g.*, in renal disease), tall, peaked T
waves, a lengthening of the P-R interval and QRS complex and a loss
of P waves occur along with a decrease in rate and force of contraction;
arrhythmias and possibly fibrillation may follow. These changes are

thought to be due to altered repolarization of the cell membrane. Potassium depletion results in tachycardia, prolongation of the P-R interval, T wave flattening and prominent U waves.

As will be described in Chapter 6, the presence of an adequate extracellular Ca^{++} concentration is essential for normal cardiac muscle contraction. At low concentrations of intra- and extracellular Ca^{++}, contraction will not take place. In animal experiments it can be shown that very high levels of extracellular Ca^{++} concentration will greatly increase the strength of cardiac contraction and if exposure is prolonged, there is less and less relaxation after each contraction until finally the heart stops in sustained calcium rigor.

ELECTROCARDIOGRAPHY

A characteristic sequence of potentials is generated by the heart muscle during each beat. Since the tissues of the body surrounding the heart are conductors of electricity, a small but constant fraction of the cardiac potentials may be picked up between two surface points (bipolar recording) and amplified and recorded. Such a graphic record is termed an *electrocardiogram* (ECG); if the electrodes are placed directly on the heart surface, the resulting trace is called an *electrogram*. A conventional method of electrocardiography is to record from electrodes on three extremities of the body, *i.e.*, left and right arms and left leg, using the right leg electrode as ground. The arrangement of these classical "limb leads" is shown graphically in Figure 5-7 (*left*). These leads were defined by Einthoven so that the major deflections in each lead would be upright (positive) in a normal subject.

The ECG is the algebraic sum of all the myocardial APs as recorded at the surface of the body. Depolarization moving toward an active electrode produces a positive deflection and if moving away, a negative one. By convention, vertical lines are spaced at 0.04-sec intervals and a paper speed of 25 mm/sec is usually employed. The vertical voltage scale is calibrated at 10 mm/mV (Fig. 5-7, *right*).

Scalar Electrocardiography—The Normal ECG

Atrial depolarization, represented by the P wave, begins at the SA node and is conducted over the atrial muscle in all directions. There are three specialized, small bundles of atrial muscle (internodal bun-

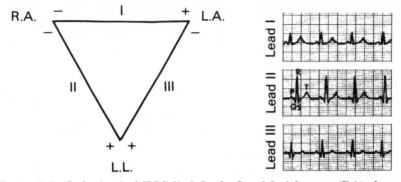

Figure 5-7. *Left*, classical ECG limb leads. *Lead I*, right arm (RA) electro-negative with respect to left arm (LA). *Lead II*, RA negative to left leg (LL) and *lead III*, LA negative to LL. *Right*, normal electrocardiogram from limb leads showing P, QRS and T waves. Wide vertical lines, 0.2 sec; narrow horizontal lines, 0.1 mV.

dles) running toward the AV node which are preferential pathways in which conduction velocity is somewhat greater. The P wave normally does not exceed 0.11 sec—which is the time for the impulse to travel over the atrium to the AV node.

At the AV node the conduction velocity slows to about 5 cm/sec, then again speeds up to velocities of 1 m/sec in the AV bundles and to about 5 m/sec in the Purkinje system before activating the ventricular muscle to contract. The time for the passage of the AP from the atrium to the ventricular muscle is called the P-R interval (Fig. 5-8). It ordinarily ranges from 0.12 to 0.21 seconds and over half of this period (from the end of the P wave to the Q wave) is taken up in transmission through the AV node. Prolongation of this interval is usually due to abnormal delay in the AV node, to bundle branch disease or to metabolic effects of chronotropic drugs such as digitalis.

Ventricular depolarization begins at the left side of the interventric-ular septum (Q wave), spreads from the endocardial to epicardial surface of the left ventricle (R wave) and finally to the right ventricle (S wave). The conduction velocity through ventricular muscle is about 0.8 to 1.0 m/sec and the width of the QRS ordinarily does not exceed 0.06 to 0.11 second. The activation times of the different parts of the heart are shown in Figure 5-1 (*right*). Ventricular repolarization pro-ceeds from epicardial to endocardial surface and is represented by the T wave. It normally takes 0.1 to 0.25 second.

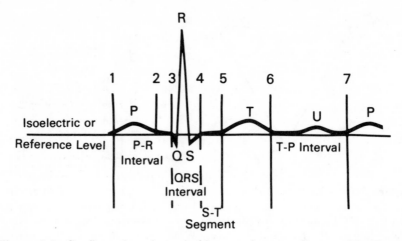

Figure 5-8. Configuration of a typical human electrocardiogram. The P wave extends from *lines 1* to *2*, the QRS from *lines 3* to *4*, the ST interval from *lines 4* to *5*, and the T wave from *lines 5* to *6*. T-P interval is the isoelectric period extending from the end of the T wave (*6*) to the beginning of the next P wave (*7*). The U wave is seen occasionally and has only minor significance.

The S-T segment is that period between the end of the QRS complex and the beginning of the T wave and represents the interval between completion of depolarization and the time when electrical recovery (repolarization) begins (Fig. 5-8). Its configuration is importantly affected by injury or ischemia of the myocardium as will be further discussed in Chapters 12 and 14. The T-P interval is an isoelectric period of quiescence whose duration varies inversely with the heart rate. The T-P interval sometimes contains a small oscillation called the U wave which is thought to represent the slow repolarization of papillary muscle; some cardiologists have reported that U wave inversion is suggestive of myocardial ischemia but otherwise the U wave has apparently little physiological or pathological significance.

Vectorcardiography—The Electrical Axis of the Heart

While the procedure described above yields a measure of the magnitude of the voltage (scalar electrocardiography) it is possible by summation to determine a resultant vector with both magnitude and direction (vectorcardiography). This is done by recording two leads simultaneously and measuring their respective voltages at the same point. Using the peak of the R wave, an example of such a determination of a resultant vector is shown in Figure 5-9.

The orientation of the resultant QRS axis in the frontal plane (the electrical axis) is usually inferior and leftward at an angle from 0° to +90°; this is in accord with the usual left ventricular predominance. If the angle is more positive, *i.e.*, rotated more rightward, it is suggestive of right ventricular preponderance (right axis deviation). Change in the electrical axis of the heart can be produced by mechanical alteration of the cardiac position and also by a wide variety of cardiac and pulmonary disorders which change the anatomical position of the heart.

Unipolar Leads

Bipolar leads, as described above, measure potential differences between two points on the surface of the body; however, they cannot

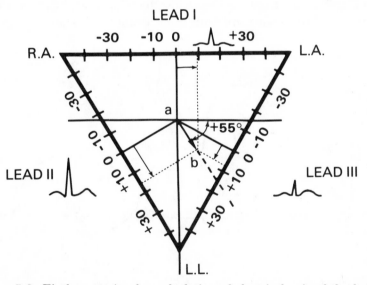

Figure 5-9. Einthoven triangle—calculation of electrical axis of the heart. Perpendiculars from the midpoint of the sides of the equilateral triangle intersect at the center of electrical activity (*a*). RA, right arm; LA, left arm; LL, left leg. If from the midpoint, distances equivalent to the wave voltage (in this case the R wave) are laid off parallel to the respective lead, perpendiculars from these end points will intersect at a point designating the magnitude and direction of the resultant R vector (*a b*).

record actual potentials at either electrode; thus waves of depolarization and repolarization at different points on the myocardium may neutralize each other and not be accurately recorded.

In 1934, Wilson introduced unipolar lead electrocardiography in which one electrode (the exploring electrode) is placed at different points on the body surface and the other, indifferent electrode, is kept at zero potential by connecting all three limbs to a central terminal through a 5000 ohm resistance. Unipolar leads are labeled V and followed by a letter or number describing the position of the exploring electrode. Because potentials so recorded may be somewhat smaller than desirable, a system of "augmented" leads is commonly used for the unipolar limb leads, *i.e.*, AVR, AVL and AVF (Fig. 5-10, *left*).

The Standard ECG

In the standard 12-lead ECG, six leads are recorded in the frontal plane and six in the transverse plane. The leads in the *frontal* plane are referred to as standard limb leads, *i.e.*, leads I, II and III and the

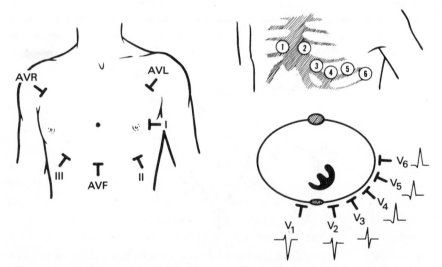

Figure 5-10. Limb leads (*left*) and precordial leads (*right*) in standard twelve-lead ECG. Limb leads include leads I, II and III and augmented limb leads with exploring electrodes on right arm (AVR), left arm (AVL) and left foot (AVF). Precordial leads V_1 to V_6 (*right*) record cardiac potentials in a transverse plane. (From R. L. DeJoseph, *Introduction to Electrocardiography: The Vectorial Approach.* East Hanover, N. J.: Sandoz Co., 1977.)

augmented limb leads, AVR, AVL and AVF. These are, in effect, positive poles of a bipolar recording system "looking at" the depolarization vectors from six different positions in the frontal plane (Fig. 5-10, *left*). The other six leads are the precordial chest leads which record the depolarization vectors in the *transverse* plane and are numbered V_1 to V_6. They are placed in positions varying from near midsternum to left midaxillary line, as shown in Figure 5-10, *right*.

In Figure 5-10 (*right*), leads V_1 to V_6 represent summation of electrical activity of both ventricles. The QRS of the left ventricle dominates because of its thicker musculature. As the excitation spreads toward the recording electrode, the deflection is positive or upward and as it moves away the deflection will be downward.

ARRHYTHMIAS

Arrhythmias are disturbances of rate, rhythm or sequence of depolarization which are due either to disorders of impulse formation or impulse conduction. Normal sinus rhythm indicates that the SA node is the pacemaker and that the rate, form and order of excitation is within normal limits. *Sinus arrhythmia*, which is common in young adults and children, refers to phasic rate changes with respiration. In sinus bradycardia the rate in the adult is by definition less than 60/min and in sinus tachycardia greater than 100/min but the rhythm, form and succession of the various ECG waves are normal.

Premature Contractions and Pathological Tachycardias

It is thought that many arrhythmias arise because of an unequal transmission velocity through branches of the conduction system with "reentry" into a proximal conduction site. The reentry theory suggests that because of ischemia or other injury there is a unidirectional block in one fiber bundle (because of partial depolarization) and a delayed or slow retrograde conduction in the previously blocked but now repolarized bundle (Fig. 5-11B). The retrograde impulse from the unblocked limb may penetrate the damaged segment, reenter, and cause a premature contraction since it has—because of the delay—reached the original pathway after the refractory period. Bidirectional block will stop the reentrant impulse (Fig. 5-11D). The process may become repetitive and result in tachycardia.

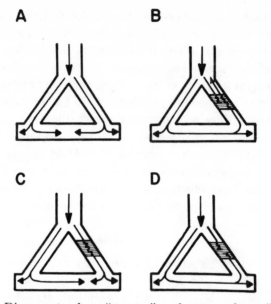

Figure 5-11. Diagram to show "reentry" pathways and possible modifications. *A*, normal velocity of propagation through Purkinje bundle branches. *B*, unidirectional (antegrade) block through a diseased branch with retrograde penetration of the depressed segment and impulse activation through reentry. The extrasystole may be suppressed by improved antegrade conduction (*C*) or development of bidirectional block (*D*). (From M. R. Rosen, B. F. Hoffman, and A. L. Wit, *Am. Heart J.* 89:526, 1975.)

In addition to disordered conduction, arrhythmias may also arise because of newly developed centers of impulse formation. All cardiac tissue may, as a result of ischemia, injury or heightened excitability, become a temporary or permanent pacemaker for the heart and thus usurp the normal pacemaker. Such sites are called "ectopic foci" and the anomolous complexes are referred to as premature or extrasystoles. These abnormal impulses may be formed in the atrium outside of the SA node (atrial premature beats), in the AV node (junctional premature beats) or in the bundle of His or ventricular muscle (ventricular ectopic beats).

The ectopic beat may also be conducted in a retrograde direction and may depolarize the SA node, atria or AV node; in this case the normal pacemaker cannot generate an impulse until repolarization is complete so that there may be an interval between beats (a compensatory pause). During this pause there will be increased ventricular filling and an increased stroke volume in the succeeding systole. The pause and the increased stroke volume are often sensed by the patient as a "skipped beat."

Atrial premature contractions result from a non-nodal atrial pacemaker and may show an abnormal P wave; there are usually normal QRS and T complexes unless there is also aberrant intraventricular conduction (Fig. 5-12, *upper*).

Ventricular extrasystoles are usually caused by an irritable or ectopic focus within the ventricle; the QRS complex may be normal but is usually abnormal (Fig. 5-12, *lower*). If the ectopic focus discharges rhythmically and thus has a constant relation to the normal QRS complex, the beat is "coupled"; if it occurs after every normal beat it is called "bigeminy" and if after every second normal beat "trigeminy" *etc.*

Paroxysmal supraventricular tachycardia occurs if the ectopic focus

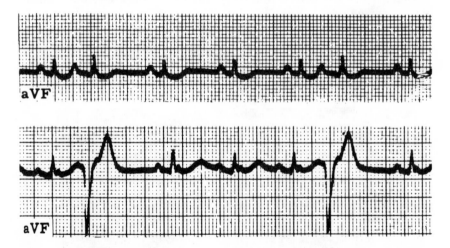

Figure 5-12. Atrial (*upper*) and ventricular (*lower*) premature contractions. *Upper*, regular sinus rhythm, rate 75/min. Normal QRS indicates that conduction through atrioventricular node and ventricles is normal. *Lower*, ventricular ectopic beats occur before completion of preceding T wave. Note aberrant QRS and no preceding P wave. (Reproduced with permission from M. J. Goldman, *Principles of Clinical Electrocardiography*, 10th ed., 1978. Copyright 1978 by Lange Medical Publications, Los Altos, Calif.)

maintains a very high atrial rate; the episodes often have a sudden onset and offset. If the rate is 250 to 300/min, the disorder becomes an atrial flutter. Flutter is a serious arrhythmia because it often has a rapid ventricular response. Either flutter or fibrillation may be followed by various degrees of heart block.

It has been suggested that atrial fibrillation results from alteration of an excitation wave so that it travels around a damaged area in a circle or "circus movement." In animal experiments, the behavior of induced atrial fibrillation is consistent with such a concept. If the ectopic focus is in the ventricle, paroxysmal ventricular tachycardia may occur (Fig. 5-13, *lower left*); this is a dangerous arrhythmia since it frequently degenerates into ventricular fibrillation (Fig. 5-13, *lower right*) in which there is complete cessation of effective ventricular contraction. Ventricular fibrillation is a common cause of sudden death.

Conduction Blocks

Blockade of the conduction path may occur anywhere between the SA node and ventricles; one of the more common sites is AV nodal block of which three degrees are usually distinguished. In first degree block all the atrial impulses reach the ventricles but the P-R interval is prolonged, *i.e.*, greater than 0.2 sec (Fig. 5-14, *upper*); this is usually due to AV junctional delay.

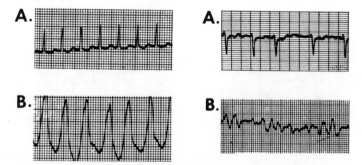

Figure 5-13. Paroxysmal atrial tachycardia (*A, left*) showing normal QRS complexes and atrial fibrillation (*A, right*) showing irregular, uncoordinated atrial waves dissociated from QRS waves. Ventricular tachycardia (*B, left*) showing rapid, abnormal QRS complexes. Ventricular fibrillation (*B, right*) shows irregular, uncoordinated QRS complexes. (From R. M. Berne and M. N. Levy, *Cardiovascular Physiology*, 3rd ed. St. Louis: C.V. Mosby Co., 1977.)

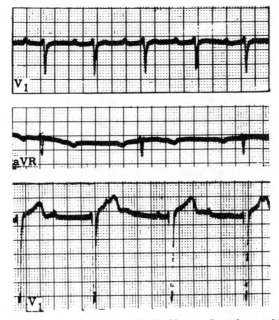

Figure 5-14. Atrioventricular heart block. *Upper*, first degree block with P-R interval of 0.28 sec but otherwise normal ECG; *middle*, second degree 2:1 block with atrial rate of 82/min and regular; ventricle responds only to every other atrial beat. *Lower*, complete heart block, atrial rate is 72/min and atria are activated by normal impulses from sinoatrial node. Ventricular rate is 54/min and independent of atrial rate. (Reproduced with permission from M. J. Goldman, *Principles of Clinical Electrocardiography*, 10th ed., 1978. Copyright 1978, Lange Medical Publications, Los Altos, Calif.)

Second degree block, in which not all the P waves are followed by QRS complexes, may be of two forms. In partial progressive AV block, the P-R interval progressively increases, culminating in a dropped beat (Wenckebach phenomenon); in the second type, the P-R interval is relatively fixed and the ratio of transmission may be 2:1, 3:1, 4:1 *etc.* A 2:1 block of the latter type is shown in Figure 5-14, *middle*.

In a third degree, complete heart block, the impulses are completely interrupted between the atria and ventricles and the QRS complexes are dissociated from the P waves (Fig. 5-14, *lower*). The ventricular rate is much slowed (usually 35 to 40/min) so that cardiac output is inadequate. Fainting often occurs because of cerebral ischemia due to the marked slowing or asystole (Stokes-Adams syndrome).

Ischemic heart disease, a common cause of arrhythmias, is discussed in Chapter 14.

Treatment of Arrhythmias

While the ECG is a most valuable diagnostic tool, it should be emphasized that it can only assess the electrical aspects of impulse generation and conduction and cannot measure cardiac contractility. A patient may have a normal ECG and yet the myocardial contractile ability may be inadequate; conversely marked ECG abnormalities may be associated with a competent heart. In diagnosis and treatment the contractile, metabolic and electrical aspects of cardiac function must all be considered.

Some disturbances such as premature beats, AV block and paroxysmal atrial tachycardia may occur without detectable structural disease of the heart. Other disorders such as second or third degree heart block, atrial flutter and fibrillation and ventricular tachycardia are usually associated with organic disorders such as metabolic or electrolyte disturbances or with cardiovascular disease such as ischemic injury or cardiomyopathy.

The treatment of arrhythmias is highly complex and requires considerable skill and judgment and only a few general principles will be discussed in this section for the purpose of pointing out the pathophysiology involved. Aside from the effort directed toward the primary cause of the disease, therapy usually involves drugs aimed at the specific cardiac disability. Inotropic agents such as digitalis glycosides which enhance the force-velocity relation of the myocardium (Chapter 6) are used to treat heart failure and will slow sinus tachycardia by improving cardiac output. Digitalis slows the heart rate partly through its vagal action and partly through direct effect on the SA node and AV node; in the latter case it slows the supraventricular tachycardia by increasing the block at the AV node. Digitalis overdosage may, however, lead to advanced AV block or tachyarrhythmias.

Antiarrhythmic agents such as quinidine and procainamide are useful in disorders such as atrial fibrillation primarily because they decrease the rate of ectopic pacemaker excitation and prolong the absolute refractory period of the atrium—thus interrupting the "circus movement."

Non-invasive methods of stimulating the vagus will sometimes abort attacks of paroxysmal atrial tachycardia; these may include carotid sinus massage, the valsalva maneuver, lateral pressure on the eyeball or the application of cool water to the face (the face immersion reflex). However, caution must be used during these procedures since strong vagal stimulation may induce asystole and carotid sinus massage occasionally results in cerebrovascular accident (stroke).

Paroxysmal atrial tachycardia is thought to be related to slow Ca^{++} influx during the plateau period of the AP; the drug verapamil, by slowing the inward Ca^{++} migration and thereby interfering with excitation-contraction coupling, can be of benefit in paroxysmal atrial tachycardia and certain arrhythmias. Lidocaine, which diminishes the automaticity of the His and Purkinje system, raises the threshold for ventricular fibrillation and causes bidirectional block in areas of conduction delay; it is often used in ventricular arrhythmias. Through its beta adrenergic blocking action, propranolol has a primary antiarrhythmic effect. It will reduce heart rate and is used to treat certain ectopic tachycardias and premature ventricular contractions.

In some cases of ectopic rhythm disorders such as atrial flutter or fibrillation, cardioversion may succeed in restoring normal rhythm. Cardioversion consists of a direct current shock applied momentarily to the chest early in systole. It temporarily depolarizes the entire heart and interrupts the circus movement of the ectopic disorder thus permitting the sinus node pacemaker to reestablish sinus rhythm.

Artificial pacemakers are often inserted in cases of heart block, Stoke-Adams syndrome and other conditions in which an inadequate heart rate is a threat to the patient. In this procedure a "demand-type," transvenous pacemaker is usually placed *via* the subclavian vein into the right ventricle. The demand, non-competitive, pacemaker releases an electrical signal (1 to 2 mA) at a rate of about 70/min only when no intrinsic cardiac impulse is sensed by the pacemaker within a preset period. Extensive experience has demonstrated the clinical usefulness of this procedure in maintaining adequate heart rate and preventing fainting attacks.

REFERENCES

BROOKS, C. M., B. F. HOFFMAN, E. E. SUCKLING, AND O. ORIAS: *Excitability of the Heart*. New York: Grune & Stratton Inc., 1955.

GOLDMAN, J. J.: *Principles of Clinical Electrocardiography*, 10th ed. Los Altos, Calif.: Lange Medical Publications, 1978.

HOFFMAN, B. F., AND P. F. CRANEFIELD: *Electrophysiology of the Heart*. New York: McGraw-Hill Book Co., 1960.

JAMES, D. G. (Ed.): *Circulation of the Blood*. Baltimore: University Park Press, 1978.

MARSHALL, J. M.: The heart. In *Medical Physiology*, ed. by V. B. Mountcastle. St. Louis: C.V. Mosby Co., 1974.

SCHER, A. M.: Electrocardiogram. In *Physiology and Biophysics*, ed. by T. C. Ruch, H. D. Patton, and A. M. Scher. Philadelphia: W. B. Saunders Co., 1974.

SCHLANT, R. C., AND J. W. HURST (Eds.): *Advances in Electrocardiography*. New York: Grune & Stratton Inc., 1972.

SOKOLOW, M., AND M. B. McILROY: *Clinical Cardiology*. Los Altos, Calif.: Lange Medical Publications, 1977.

TRAUTWEIN, W.: Generation and conduction of impulses in the heart as affected by drugs. *Pharmacol. Rev.* 15:277, 1963.

WILSON, F. N., F. D. JOHNSON, A. G. McLEOD, AND P. S. BARKER: Electrocardiograms that represent the potential variations of a single electrode. *Am. Heart J.* 9:447, 1934.

chapter 6

Contractile Properties of the Heart

STRUCTURAL AND FUNCTIONAL CHARACTERISTICS OF THE MYOFIBRIL

The muscle fiber is composed of myofibrils which on microscopic section show longitudinal strands of thick myosin and thin actin filaments. The basic structural unit is the sarcomere, that portion between the Z lines (Fig. 6-1).

Contraction of the myocardial fiber involves a complex series of chemical and physical events. The essential process consists of chemical activation by Ca^{++} of the proteins of the actin and myosin filaments and of the cross bridges which run between them. As a result the myosin and actin filaments interdigitate and slide upon each other (sliding filament hypothesis), pulling the Z lines toward each other, thus shortening and contracting the muscle.

Essential to this process is the rapid influx of Ca^{++} ions across the sarcolemmal membrane and the release of Ca^{++} from intracellular sites

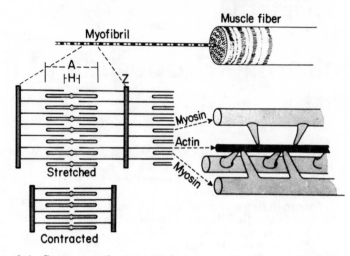

Figure 6-1. Structure of myocardial muscle cell. The myofibrils consist of overlapping thick myosin and thin actin filaments with cross bridges between them. As shown diagrammatically (*right*) the cross bridges form linkages at specific sites on the actin fibers, pulling the actin filament lengthwise to contract the muscle. (From R. Rushmer, *Structure and Function of Cardiovascular System*. Philadelphia: W. B. Saunders Co., 1976.)

by means of excitation-contraction coupling. Essentially, such coupling involves depolarization of the transverse (T) tubules and release of Ca^{++} from storage sites within the sarcoplasmic reticulum (Fig. 6-2).

Small sac-like expansions of the sarcoplasmic reticulum, called subsarcolemmal cisternae (Fig. 6-2) are located near the Z lines. The three units—the longitudinal superficial sarcoplasmic reticulum, the transverse system (T tubes) and the cisternae are closely involved in the contraction-relaxation sequence.

EXCITATION-CONTRACTION COUPLING

The ionic and electrical aspects of the cardiac action potential (AP) were described in Chapter 5. Although the exact relationship between the AP and muscle contraction is not fully understood, the intracellular mobilization of Ca^{++} in adequate quantities in its so-called "activator" state undoubtedly plays a pivotal role. This is shown by the fact that at low concentrations of extracellular Ca^{++}, the AP will not elicit a contraction. Furthermore, the contractile process necessitates an influx

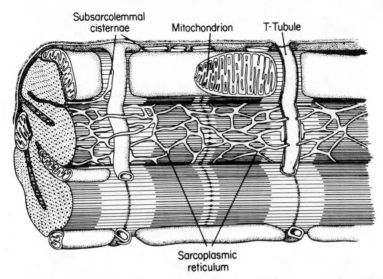

Figure 6-2. Myofibril showing sarcoplasmic reticulum. The muscle fibril is enveloped by a cell membrane which has tubular projections (T or transverse tubules) which are open to the extracellular space. A second completely intracellular membrane system, *i.e.*, the sarcoplasmic reticulum, makes close contact with the T tubules and sarcolemma. (From W. Bloom and D. W. Fawcett, *Textbook of Histology.* Philadelphia: W. B. Saunders Co., 1969.)

of Ca^{++} and the resultant strength of contraction is directly correlated with the extracellular Ca^{++} concentration.

The combination of Ca^{++} with the muscle proteins is a key factor in excitation-contraction coupling; aside from actin and myosin, the thin filaments of the myofibril contain at least two other proteins, *viz.*, tropomyosin and the "troponin complex"; a suggested interrelationship of these elements is shown schematically in Figure 6-3.

During the plateau of the AP there is an influx of extracellular Ca^{++} into the cell and also a release of previously bound Ca^{++} from intracellular stores, primarily in the sarcoplasmic reticulum and cisternae. The combination of the "activator" Ca^{++} with troponin complex results in the removal of an inhibitory effect of tropomysin, permitting attachment of myosin bridges to sites on the actin filament. Subsequent hydrolysis of the terminal phosphate on ATP supplies the chemical energy required for generation of a mechanical force at each cross-bridge attachment. The conversion is mediated by flexion of the cross

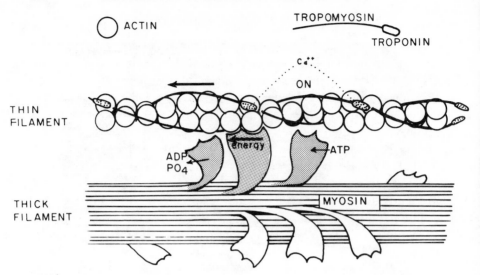

Figure 6-3. Schema illustrating elements concerned in cardiac muscle contraction. The actin filament is closely bound to two additional proteins, *i.e.*, tropomyosin and troponin complex. During the plateau of the action potential, Ca^{++} ions bind with troponin which triggers the coupling of actin and myosin and the movement of the cross bridges. Pulled by the cross bridges, the filaments slide across each other, pulling the Z lines together and causing contraction. (After R. Rushmer, *Structure and Function of the Cardiovascular System.* Philadelphia: W. B. Saunders Co., 1976.)

bridge and interdigitation of the filaments with consequent contraction of the muscle fiber. After the plateau phase of the AP and repolarization of the cell membrane, the intracellular Ca^{++} is again bound to the sarcoplasmic reticulum or extruded from the cell.

Thus the AP through its regulation of the intracellular concentration of activator Ca^{++}, not only triggers the contraction but influences its magnitude and duration. The force of contraction appears to depend on the number of cross bridges formed and this number is related to the intracellular Ca^{++} concentration. Inotropic agents may act at several possible sites. Catecholamines appear to act by increasing the intracellular concentration of cyclic AMP and thus of available energy for the cross linkage. The site of action of digitalis is not certain; it has been suggested that by inhibiting the Na^+ pump action it facilitates the entry of Ca^{++} during the AP.

ELASTIC PROPERTIES OF THE MYOCARDIUM

Heart muscle possesses elastic as well as contractile properties. If a strip of myocardium is passively elongated it will develop tension disproportionate to the applied stretch. It is advantageous for conceptual purposes to separate the contractile and elastic elements of cardiac muscle; compliance (elasticity), *e.g.*, is an important factor in determining the resistance to diastolic inflow into the ventricle and ultimately, therefore, in determining stroke volume.

The elastic components of myocardium have been visualized by some investigators as separate parallel and series elements as shown in Figure 6-4.

The parallel element, PE, (Fig. 6-4) represents the elastic behavior of resting muscle and SE the elastic behavior of contracting muscle. CE represents all the contractile elements. When muscle first contracts, shortening is rapid because the resisting load is small but as shortening develops in isotonic contraction, the SE lengthens and with the tension increase, the velocity of contraction decreases. The force registered at the ends of the muscle will depend, therefore, not only on the contractile properties of CE, but on the elastic properties of SE and the time allowed for interaction between the lengthening of SE and shortening of CE. It should be emphasized that this concept is a

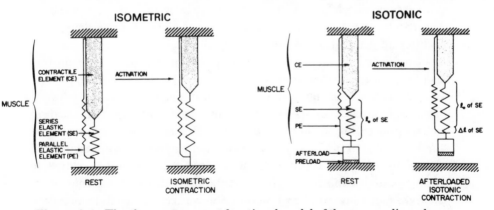

Figure 6-4. The three-component functional model of the myocardium showing the contractile component (CE), parallel elastic component (PE) and series elastic component (SE). CE and SE are in series with each other and PE is parallel with them. The elastic elements are passive springs and the contractile element is freely extensible. (From E. H. Sonnenblick, *Fed. Proc.* 21:975, 1962.)

theoretical one useful for analytical purposes. No anatomical analogues actually exist as purely contractile or elastic elements.

MYOCARDIAL CONTRACTILITY

How well the heart can propel blood is unquestionably the greatest single determinant of circulatory performance. But what factors regulate myocardial contractility and how to measure it are questions which still provoke frequent debates and sharply dissenting views among investigators. In the following, emphasis will be placed on those aspects which seem most relevant to cardiac function in the intact human.

The strength of cardiac contraction can be influenced in two general ways: (a) through alteration of diastolic filling, *i.e.*, change in precontractile length of the muscle, which is an intrinsic regulatory process; or (b) by altering its inotropic or contractile state, which is an extrinsic effect, usually brought about by neural or hormonal influences.

Intrinsic Regulation of the Myocardium

A. Diastolic Filling—Starling's Law of the Heart. This very basic concept, originally described by Frank and Starling, states in effect that within physiological limits, the force or tension generated by the contracting muscle is greater if the muscle is previously stretched. This can be shown by determining *in vitro* the peak tension developed at different precontractile lengths (Fig. 6-5).

As indicated in Figure 6-5, not only the time to peak tension but also the time to relaxation was unchanged when fiber length was altered. This would imply that if, in the intact heart, there is during diastole a greater influx of blood into the ventricle, the ensuing contraction will then be more forceful. This may be thought of as a "preload" stimulus since it was applied before contraction began.

Starling, an English physiologist, studied this phenomenon further in an isolated, canine heart-lung preparation in which he controlled the right atrial pressure (and thereby the ventricular diastolic pressure or preload) by raising or lowering an infusion bottle connected to the vena cava; he also controlled the aortic pressure (or afterload) by means of an artificial aortic resistance. From a series of such experiments Starling showed that with increased diastolic volume, the sub-

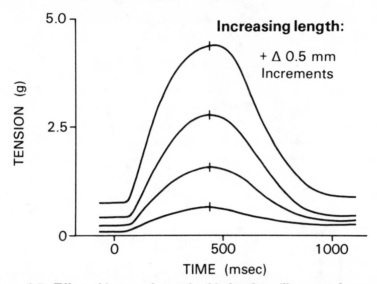

Figure 6-5. Effect of increased stretch of isolated papillary muscle on contractile force showing isometric contractions of the isolated muscle at different precontractile lengths while using stimuli of the same strength. Note that while the generated tension increases progressively, the time to maximal tension is constant. (From E. H. Sonnenblick, *Fed. Proc.* 21:975, 1962.)

sequent contraction of the isolated heart did indeed result in a higher peak systolic pressure; his data also showed that if the ventricle is stretched beyond the physiological limit, the systolic pressure will decline, indicating impending failure (Fig. 6-6).

Sarnoff and Mitchell found that similar relationships exist between left ventricular end-diastolic pressure (LVEDP) and LV stroke work; because the length-tension relationship of the two ventricles are usually comparable, graphs depicting *right* ventricular volume and *left* ventricular pressure—as was done originally by Starling—also show similar configurations.

This characteristic of the myocardium—also called "heterometric autoregulation"—is an inherent, intrinsic property of the muscle fiber which is evident in the heart fully isolated from all neural or humoral influences. It has been suggested that this property is due to the apposition—as the muscle is stretched—of more cross bridges between the actin and myosin; it was further theorized that the "failure" part

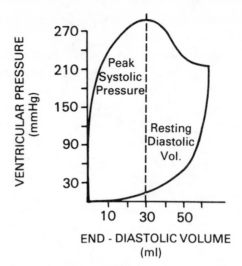

Figure 6-6. Starling volume-pressure curve of myocardial function. Classical curve indicating that within physiological limits, increased end-diastolic ventricular volume will result in increased peak ventricular pressure. Beyond the *dotted lines* the ventricle is overstretched and the heart will respond to increased filling with less pressure. (From S. W. Patterson, H. Pipers, and E. H. Starling, *J. Physiol.* 48:465, 1914.)

of the curve occurs because sarcomeres are stretched beyond their normal length of about 2.2 μm and that fewer cross bridges are thereby formed between the filaments.

However, in a recent study of heart failure in dogs, investigators did not find increases in sarcomere lengths and expressed the belief that the reduced contractility of the failing myocardium is related to an intrinsic defect of the muscle rather than to its position on the descending limb of the Starling curve. Further evidence is needed on this question.

The Starling effect is an important one, however, since it enables the heart to adapt its pumping capacity to alterations in venous return. The contractile response to altered myocardial length is particularly helpful in matching the output of the two ventricles and thus keeping the pulmonary and systemic systems in balance.

Aside from precontractile length, two other intrinsic factors, *i.e.*, interval-strength effects and homeometric autoregulation may, under certain circumstances, influence myocardial contraction.

B. Interval-Strength Effects. Heart rate will influence stroke volume through its temporal effect on diastolic filling time (Chapter 7). But there are additional intrinsic "interval-strength" factors which can produce temporary alterations in myocardial contractility. Interval-strength relationships are complex and only three effects will be considered here. A rapid rate increase will, for the next few beats, progressively augment cardiac contractility—the staircase or "treppe" phenomenon (Fig. 6-7, *left*).

Similarly, a delay between beats or a pause after an extrasystole (post extrasystolic potentiation) will be followed by stronger contractions; these effects, which are clearly intrinsic and not dependent on increased filling, are nonetheless amplified in the intact heart by the added mechanical effect of increased diastolic filling. The interval-strength relation, which is of relatively minor importance in the normal intact human, is probably due to a time-induced alteration in Ca^{++} availability to the muscle cell.

C. Homeometric Autoregulation. As will be discussed later in this chapter, increase in afterload will cause a decrease in strength, velocity and duration of contraction of the isolated heart muscle; similarly, increase in aortic pressure will cause comparable effects in the intact ventricle (Chapter 7). However, in certain instances, particularly in anesthetized animals after abrupt increase in aortic pressure, there may be an initial decrease followed by a temporary *elevation* of strokework. This is not a mechanical but apparently an intrinsic, inotropic

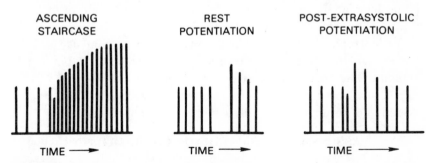

Figure 6-7. Myocardial contraction: The interval-strength relation. An increase in heart rate, a prolonged beat interval and a delay after an extrasystole all result in stronger subsequent contractions. (From E. O. Feigl, *Physiology and Biophysics*, ed. by T. C. Ruch and H. D. Patton. Philadelphia: W. B. Saunders Co., 1974.)

response of the myocardium; it is known as the "Anrep" effect or "homeometric autoregulation" since it occurs without any change in fiber length. Existing evidence suggests that this phenomenon probably plays only a minor role in myocardial contraction in the intact human circulation.

Extrinsic Regulation of the Myocardium—Inotropic State

Outside factors which affect the inotropic state or contractility of the heart may be of three general types: (A) *neurohormonal effects*, due to influences of the sympathetic or parasympathetic systems or of the catecholamines; (B) *chemical and pharmacological effects*, e.g., contractile changes due to alterations in blood K^+, Ca^{++} or pH, or to drugs such as digitalis and sympathetic "blockers"; and (C) *pathological effects*, e.g., those due to ischemia incident to coronary occlusion or toxic effects resulting from bacteria or chemicals.

These extrinsic factors all exert their inotropic effect by altering ventricular pressure or stroke work without a change in diastolic length; thus at equivalent end-diastolic volumes, higher (or lower) ventricular pressures will be elaborated (Fig. 6-8).

As shown in Figure 6-8, sympathetic stimulation will produce a positive inotropic effect and move the Starling curve upward and to the left depending on the strength of stimulation; increased contractility will also result from injection of norepinephrine, digitalis or Ca^{++} ions. Conversely myocardial ischemia, toxic and anesthetic agents, hypocalcemia, hyperpotassemia, or cardiac failure will result in a negative inotropic effect and a lowered curve.

The inotropic effects are probably related to their influence on Ca^{++} delivery to the contractile sites and to the rate of Ca^{++} binding to troponin. The normal serum calcium concentration (about 4.3 to 5.3 mEq/L) is about 10,000 times that of the myocardial cell; yet a reduction of serum calcium will lessen myocardial contractility.

ASSESSMENT OF CARDIAC CONTRACTILITY

As described above, in the intact human circulation, the strength of cardiac contraction may be altered in two primary ways: (a) by altering diastolic filling, *i.e.*, changing precontractile muscle length, an intrinsic effect; or (b) by altering the inotropic state or contractility, an extrinsic effect.

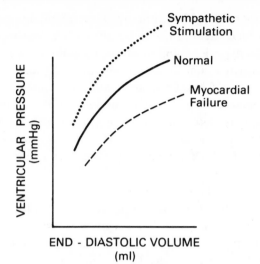

Figure 6-8. Effect of sympathetic stimulation and pathological changes on myocardial contractility. Sympathetic stimulation or administration of nor-epinephrine or digitalis will move the Starling curve up and to the left and improve ventricular function—a positive inotropic effect. With myocardial ischemia, toxic agents or heart failure, the curve is moved down and to the right and there is a lesser ventricular pressure produced at the same end—diastolic filling volume—a negative inotropic effect.

But in evaluating cardiac function, a distinction should be made between "performance" and "contractility." Cardiac performance refers to measurements such as stroke volume and cardiac output which depend on contractility but are also influenced by mechanical or other extraneous factors. Contractility is the more important measurement and refers to a careful estimate, under controlled conditions, of the basic ability of the heart muscle to generate power. Circulatory performance such as cardiac output may, for example, be adversely affected by decreased blood volume or an incompetent valve while the contractile ability of the myocardium may be entirely normal.

This distinction would be an important one for instance after a myocardial infarct, when it would be helpful to have a quantitative measure of the remaining myocardial contractile ability so that an estimate might be made as to whether the patient may be an acceptable risk for myocardial revascularization surgery.

There are four major determinants of myocardial performance, *i.e.*, preload, afterload, heart rate and contractility (inotropic state). As previously noted, preload and inotropic capability are major determinants of myocardial contractile power while afterload and heart rate (to be discussed in Chapter 7) are mainly mechanical factors which affect performance. By maintaining preload, afterload and heart rate constant, one may determine the effect of drugs, catecholamines or other interventions on contractility. Alternatively, one may maintain the heart rate, afterload and extrinsic factors constant and determine the effect of preload.

While such procedures are possible with cardiac muscle strips or isolated heart preparations, they are usually difficult or impossible in the intact organism. Methods have been designed to approximate this ideal and to estimate myocardial contractility in the intact subject but none is as yet fully satisfactory. Among the more widely used methods are (a) the measurement of contraction velocity (force-velocity curves) and (b) the determination of maximum rate of rise of left ventricular pressure (dP/dt max). In addition to these two measures, some investigators have recently suggested that the ventricular ejection fraction (EF), *i.e.*, the ratio of stroke volume to end-diastolic volume (described in Chapter 14) may provide a clinically useful index of cardiac contractility.

Force-Velocity Curves

If a cardiac muscle strip is made to lift a load after contraction has begun (afterloading), the muscle gradually develops tension as the series elastic element (Fig. 6-4) is stretched, so that after a brief interval the muscle begins to shorten. At first the velocity of shortening is high but as the elastic tension rises, the velocity gradually diminishes. When the afterload is increased in steps, the degree of shortening, the velocity of shortening and the total time of contraction all decrease. (Fig. 6-9, *lower left*).

The counterpart of this in the intact human is the decreased stroke volume, decreased ejection velocity and shortened ejection time when the aortic pressure rises (Chapter 7); the myocardial fibers need a longer time to develop the tension required to overcome the greater afterload. At the lightest load, the initial velocity of contraction is greatest. If the velocities are plotted against afterload (Fig. 6-9, *right*),

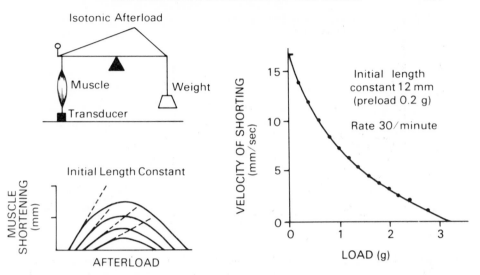

Figure 6-9. Influence of afterload on velocity and degree of shortening of myocardium. When a muscle is permitted to shorten (isotonic contraction) against different afterloads (*upper left*), the degree of shortening and initial velocity (- - -) decrease as afterload is increased (*lower left*). The plot of force (afterload) *vs* and initial velocity of shortening with different afterloads is shown at the right. At 3.1 *g*, the load is too heavy to lift, the velocity is zero and the contraction is isometric. (After E. H. Sonnenblick, *Fed. Proc.* 21:975, 1962.)

the velocity curve extrapolated to the y axis would represent the velocity at zero load, *i.e.*, maximum velocity (V_{max}).

In the above experiment, the initial muscle length (preload) was held constant and the afterload varied. If now, the preload is varied, *i.e.*, the muscle stretched to a larger precontractile length and the muscle again subjected to different afterloads, curves similar to those of Figure 6-10 (*left*) will result.

It will be noted in Figure 6-10 (*left*) that the muscle with the greater preload (and thereby stretched) can overcome a larger afterload, which is in accord with Starling's law; but in addition, it is significant that V_{max} in the two cases is the same, *i.e.*, V_{max} is independent of preload. If now norepinephrine or Ca^{++} ions are added to the isolated muscle, or if the sympathetic nerves to the intact heart are stimulated, the force-velocity curve is moved upward and to the right and V_{max} is increased (Fig. 6-10, *right*). Thus a stronger myocardial contraction

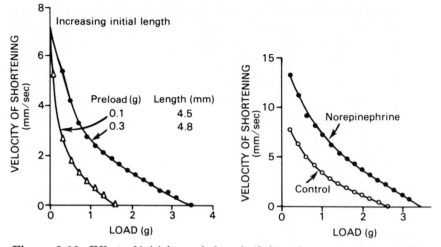

Figure 6-10. Effect of initial muscle length (*left*) and norepinephrine (*right*) on force-velocity curve of myocardial contraction. While a greater preload shifts the curve to the right, maximum velocity (V_{max}) of contraction is unchanged (*left*). Positive inotropic agents such as norepinephrine or sympathetic stimulators move the curve to the right and increase V_{max}. (From E. H. Sonnenblick, *Fed. Proc.* 21:975, 1962.)

may result through an improved ventricular volume-pressure (Starling) effect (Fig. 6-6 or 6-10, *left*) or by increased velocity of shortening and increased V_{max}, extrinsically induced (Fig. 6-10, *right*).

V_{max} has been used as an inotropic index in isolated muscle and heart preparations, but the achievement of graded afterloads under controlled conditions is difficult in intact hearts. V_{max} has been estimated in the normally beating heart using the isovolumic phase of contraction. Complex three-dimensional analyses of force, velocity and length have also been made in an effort to achieve a single measure of contractility which incorporates all three variables; these procedures are, however, still in the investigative stage. While there is not full agreement as to its validity, V_{max} and the force-velocity concept have provided greater insight into myocardial dynamics.

Ventricular Pressure Rise (Left Ventricular dP/dt Max)

In this method, sensitive manometers are used to record the ventricular pressure curve; the tangent of the steepest point of the curve (or the peak of a wave recorded by a differentiating circuit) indicates the maximum rate of pressure change. This occurs during the isovolumic phase and is a reasonable index of the initial velocity of myocardial contraction (Fig. 6-11).

Although dP/dt max will vary to some extent with preload and heart rate, it is very responsive to changes in the inotropic state and has been used clinically to characterize the contractile ability of the heart. The left ventricular dP/dt max, which is normally about 1600 mm Hg/sec, tends to be less than 1200 mm Hg/sec in patients with disorders of the left ventricular myocardium. One of the problems with this determination is a technical one, *i.e.*, even with high fidelity, catheter-tip manometers which eliminate much of the distortion of the pressure wave due to fluid transmission through the catheter, recording artefacts are still difficult to avoid.

Considerable effort is currently being expended in the search for

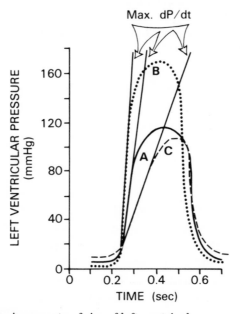

Figure 6-11. Maximum rate of rise of left ventricular pressure (peak dP/dt). Left ventricular pressure curves with the tangent at the steepest part of ascending limb designating maximum dP/dt. *A*, control; *B*, after norepinephrine; and *C*, cardiac failure. (From R. M. Berne and M. N. Levy, *Cardiovascular Physiology*, p. 85. St. Louis: C.V. Mosby Co., 1977.)

useful, non-invasive methods for assessing cardiac performance and contractility. Some of these are discussed further in Chapter 7.

REFERENCES

BRAUNWALD, E., J. ROSS, AND E. H. SONNENBLICK: *Mechanisms of Contraction of the Normal and Failing Heart*, 2nd ed. Boston: Little, Brown & Co., 1976.

LANGER, G. A., J. S. FRANK, AND A. J. BRADY: The myocardium. In *Cardiovascular Physiology II*, vol. 9, International Review of Physiology, ed. by A. C. Guyton and A. W. Cowley. Baltimore: University Park Press, 1976.

LEVY, M. N., AND R. M. BERNE: Heart. *Annu. Rev. Physiol.* 32:373, 1970.

RANDALL, W. C.: *Neural Regulation of the Heart*, New York: Oxford University Press, 1977.

ROSS, J., JR., E. H. SONNENBLICK, R. R. TAYLOR, H. M. SPOTNITZ, AND J. W. COVELL: Diastolic geometry and sarcomere length in the chronically dilated canine left ventricle. *Circ. Res.* 28:49, 1971.

SARNOFF, S. J.: Myocardial contractility as described by ventricular function curves. *Physiol. Rev.* 35:107, 1955.

SONNENBLICK, E.: Force-velocity relations in mammalian heart muscle. *Am. J. Physiol.* 202:931, 1962.

STARLING, E. H.: *The Linacre Lecture on the Law of the Heart.* London: Longmans, Green & Co., 1918.

chapter **7**

Venous Return and Cardiac Output

Undoubtedly the most important single cardiovascular variable is the output of the heart. It is usually defined as the quantity of blood ejected by either ventricle per minute and since the two ventricles, except in unusual circumstances, are in balance, the two outputs are generally equal. In the resting human adult, mean flow to the entire body (tissue flow) is about 70 ml/kg/min so that total flow or cardiac output in an average sized subject (70 kg) is about 5 L/min. The two

113

prime determinants of tissue blood flow are its mass and metabolic rate. However, for reasons not entirely clear, cardiac output correlates slightly better with surface area than with mass; using the former as a basis, the average output value, called the *cardiac index*, is about 3.2 L/min/m^2 body surface.

REGULATION OF CARDIAC OUTPUT—GENERAL

In a closed, artificial, hydraulic system consisting of a pump and pipes, the output depends on the characteristics of the pump, of the system and of the fluid. To obtain any required flow, the usual procedure is to determine the resistance, and then set the pump speed at the level necessary to overcome that resistance and thus achieve the desired pressure and output.

In the human circulation, however, the situation is quite different; the pipe system and the fluid are able to change characteristics from time to time and thereby impose varying demands on the pump. On the other hand, the pump has, in its own right, a wide latitude in altering its own characteristics in order to meet these demands.

As will be discussed in Chapter 9, the overriding determinant of total flow in any organism of fixed mass is the metabolic rate; as a consequence, flow requirements will rise markedly in fever or exercise and decrease in conditions such as sleep or hypothyroidism. But these changes in output are induced by metabolic requirements of the body and not by switching the pump to a different setting; in other words it is the body which sets the pace and not the pump.

Thus from a flow standpoint, the heart plays a "permissive" role and does not regulate its own output. So in the human circulation, the heart functions as a "demand" pump and will eject only the minimum volume demanded of it. The healthy, normal heart does, however, have impressive resources at its own disposal and is well able to meet a large range of ordinary demands; nevertheless, when diseased, the heart becomes the limiting factor in controlling the output and when it cannot cope, signs and symptoms of failure appear (Chapter 14).

For these reasons it is necessary to consider the regulation of cardiac output from two different standpoints: (a) *the role of systemic factors* in determining cardiac output, which means, in effect, what influences the return of blood to the heart; and (b) *the role of cardiac factors* in determining cardiac output, *i.e.*, what influences the ability of the heart to meet altered demands.

SYSTEMIC FACTORS DETERMINING CARDIAC OUTPUT— VENOUS RETURN CURVES

In Chapter 4 in a discussion of venous flow, it was emphasized that the primary factor influencing return of blood to the heart was the force transmitted by left ventricular ejection through the arteries to the veins. This pressure gradient, which is sometimes called the "vis a tergo" (force from behind), has been termed by Guyton the systemic filling pressure (P_{SF}). Guyton further suggested that the P_{SF}, which is $P_{SF} = P_{mc}$ the mean circulatory pressure from the root of the aorta to the vena cavae, can be determined by suddenly arresting the heart and permitting rapid equalization of pressures between the arterial and venous circuits.

Determined in this manner, the P_{SF} is about 7 mm Hg in the dog 7 mm Hg and is believed to be very similar to this in man. The difference between the P_{SF}—the mean driving pressure—and the right atrial pressure (P_{RA}) will then be the net pressure gradient determining the actual venous return. Under circumstances in which nervous and other controls are not operative, the venous return can theoretically be predicted from curves showing the respective P_{SF}s and P_{RA}s (Fig. 7-1).

In the schema of Figure 7-1, the estimated venous return can be read off the y axis at the intersecting point of the P_{RA} and P_{SF} curve. At normal values of 7 mm Hg P_{SF} and about zero for P_{RA}, the 7 mm gradient will induce a venous flow of about 5.5 L/min. In case of decreased blood volume (*e.g.*, hemorrhage) or loss of sympathetic tone, which would decrease both arterial and venous pressure, the P_{SF} will also decrease; if the P_{SF} decreases to 5.2 and P_{RA} remains constant, the net pressure gradient would be reduced to 5.2 and venous return will decrease to about 4 L/min. If the P_{SF} is 7 and P_{RA} is increased to 2 mm Hg, the output will also be reduced to about 4 L/min. Increased venous return curves, *e.g.*, the above-normal P_{SF} curve of 10.5 mm Hg in Figure 7-1 might occur with increased blood volume, increased sympathetic stimulation or a massive contraction of skeletal muscle with excessive skeletal muscle pump action and heightened peripheral venous pressure.

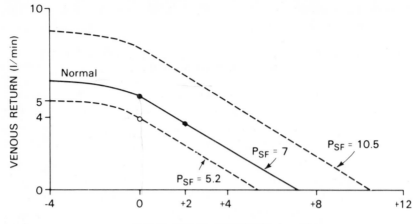

Figure 7-1. On the normal venous return curve (solid line), the venous return is about 5.5 L/min when the systemic filling pressure (P_{SF}) is 7 mm and the right atrial pressure (P_{RA}) about 0. If on the normal curve, the P_{RA} is increased to about 2 mm Hg or the P_{SF} decreased to 5.2 mm Hg, the venous return would decrease to about 4 L/min. (From A. C. Guyton, *Circulatory Physiology: Cardiac Output and Its Regulation.* Philadelphia: W. B. Saunders Co., 1973.)

It will be noted that the P_{SF} curves become flat at right atrial pressures below the zero level. This plateau is due to the collapse of veins entering the chest whenever the transmural pressure is less than zero. This stops effective flow no matter what the right atrial-P_{SF} gradient may be.

While the venous return curves involve certain abstractions and include parameters which are difficult to measure, Guyton's analytic approach has been of considerable theoretical and practical assistance in understanding the basic factors concerned with venous return. This concept also permits a combination of venous return and cardiac output curves into a single graph (Fig. 7-2). In Figure 7-2A are shown normal venous return and cardiac output values in which these two variables are both related to right atrial pressure. The two curves intersect at a value of 5 L/min (point *a*). If the blood volume is increased by transfusion, the P_{SF} will be considerably increased as will the venous return and cardiac output (point *b*).

Sympathetic stimulation has two effects; it will (a) constrict the peripheral vessels, increase the P_{SF} and, therefore, venous return, and

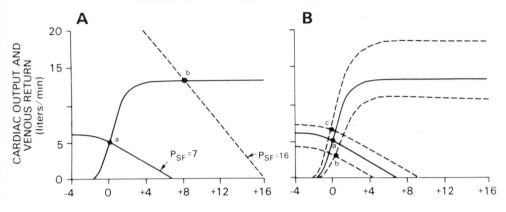

Figure 7-2. Venous return and cardiac output curves. *A*, a large blood transfusion increases the systemic filling pressure (P_{SF}) from 7 to 16 mm Hg and the right atrial pressure from 0 to 8 mm Hg. As a result, the venous return is considerably increased, *i.e.*, from point *a* to point *b*. *B*, sympathetic stimulation increases P_{SF} through contraction of peripheral vessels and so moves the venous return curve from the *solid line* to the *upper dashed line*; simultaneously it increases ventricular contractility and shifts the atrial pressure-cardiac output curve to the left. The cardiac output is, therefore, moved from point *a* to point *c*. Conversely, with sympathetic inhibition, the cardiac output might be reduced from point *a* to *b*. (From A. C. Guyton, *Circulatory Physiology: Cardiac Output and Its Regulation.* Philadelphia: W. B. Saunders Co., 1973.)

(b) increase cardiac contractile strength (Chapter 6) which will move the cardiac output curve to the left; with sympathetic stimulation as shown in Figure 7-2*B*, the venous return and cardiac output would both increase and their junction point would move from point *a* to *c*. Decreased sympathetic activity will have the reverse effect and move the cardiac output from point *a* to *b*.

It should be emphasized that the responses to some of the stresses described above such as increased blood volume, hemorrhage and sympathetic stimulation, are those which occur in a living system if no corrective measures ensue. The fact is that the hemodynamic responses to such shifts of volumes and pressures are ordinarily damped by autonomic circulatory reflexes (Chapter 10) with a gradual return to the normal state. However, an understanding of the initial tendencies is important because they may persist for appreciable periods of time and in the diseased state, may even progress.

CARDIAC FACTORS DETERMINING CARDIAC OUTPUT

Since the heart is a demand pump, it must be able to make moment by moment adjustments in order to cope (a) with shifting preload requirements of the body as manifested by alterations in venous return, and (b) with sudden circulatory changes which may arise as a result of stress and which require rapid changes in output. Since cardiac output is the product of stroke volume (SV) and heart rate (HR), such adjustments may be made by alteration in either or both of these two parameters.

At a HR of 70/min the SV of a normal resting adult will be approximately 70 to 80 ml. The mean end-diastolic volume (EDV) at rest is variable but will normally range from about 110 to 130 ml. The ejection fraction (EF), *i.e.*, the ratio of SV/EDV, is normally about 67% in man but somewhat lower (45 to 65%) in the faster beating canine heart; the blood remaining after ejection is called the end-systolic volume (ESV). The EDV and ESV can be considered, in a sense, as reserve stroke volume.

In the supine position, central blood volume, atrial filling pressure and EDV are all relatively high; with exercise in the supine position, SV is increased mainly by more complete ventricular emptying, *i.e.*, by using systolic reserve and decreasing ESV (Fig. 7-3A). In the erect

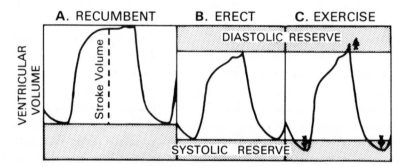

Figure 7-3. Reserve stroke volume. Schematic representation showing ventricular volume and stroke volume (SV). Upon standing, heart rate is increased and stroke volume decreased; with exercise in the erect position, SV is increased through encroachment on both diastolic and systolic reserve. (Adapted from R. F. Rushmer, *Cardiovascular Dynamics.* Philadelphia: W. B. Saunders Co., 1976.)

position, HR is increased, atrial filling pressure, EDV and SV are all decreased (Fig. 7-3*B*). Upon exercise in the erect position, HR is further increased and SV is increased by both a greater diastolic filling with increased EDV, and a more complete systolic emptying and decreased ESV (Fig. 7-3*C*).

Regulation of Stroke Volume

The four primary factors described in Chapter 6 as determinants of myocardial performance are also the main determinants of stroke volume; these factors are *diastolic filling (heterometric autoregulation), inotropic state (contractility), aortic pressure (afterload)* and the *heart rate.* The first two of these factors importantly affect myocardial contraction; the last two exert mainly mechanical effects on cardiac output.

A. Diastolic Filling. As described in Chapter 6, the heart has an important intrinsic capability enabling it to make adjustments to changes in EDV. With increased venous return and increased filling, there is increased strength of the subsequent contraction and increased stroke volume; with decreased filling the reverse occurs.

B. Inotropic State. This important extrinsic factor enables the heart to contract more strongly at an equivalent diastolic volume. In the normal circulation, a positive inotropic effect is commonly mediated through sympathoadrenal discharge which will improve cardiac performance in several ways, *viz.*, ventricular contraction is more rapid (increased V_{max} and dP/dt) and is stronger. As a result the ventricles empty more completely, *i.e.*, there is a decreased ESV and increased SV, which will produce higher systolic pressures in the ventricle and aorta. Diastolic compliance, however, is not affected. If the cause of the increased inotropic state is sympathetic stimulation, there will be an associated increase in heart rate; as discussed below, the degree of stroke volume increase may be limited by the shortening of ventricular filling time incident to the rate increase. However, with sympathetic stimulation, the net result is usually an increased cardiac output. A negative inotropic effect, by vagal stimulation, will decrease heart rate and impulse conduction and diminish atrial contractility.

C. Aortic Pressure (Afterload). Alteration of aortic pressure will produce important effects on cardiac function because of the mechanical resistance it imposes on left ventricular emptying. Such aortic pressure changes, which are suddenly presented to the left ventricle when the aortic valve opens, will result in reciprocal changes in strength, velocity and duration of left ventricular ejection and stroke volume. These effects were discussed in Chapter 6 and shown in the isolated cardiac muscle in Figure 6-9. In the intact animal, as shown in Figure 7-4, there is, at the same atrial pressure, an inverse relation between aortic pressure and stroke volume.

    D. Effect of Heart Rate on Stroke Volume. At a constant left atrial filling pressure, an increase in heart rate will decrease the diastolic filling time, and consequently, through heterometric autoregulation, will decrease stroke volume. Ventricular filling occurs mainly during

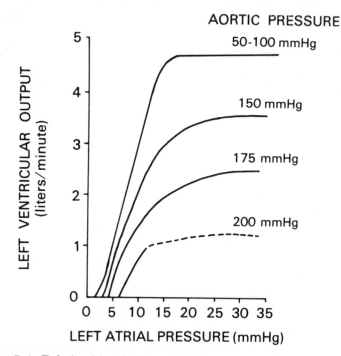

Figure 7-4. Relationship of left ventricular output and aortic pressure. As aortic pressure is increased, the left ventricular output decreases at the same left atrial pressures. The heart rate was constant so that the afterload effect was on the stroke volume. (From K. Sagawa, *Physical Bases of Circulatory Transport: Regulation and Exchange.* Philadelphia: W. B. Saunders Co., 1967.)

the rapid filling phases. A modest increase in heart rate will encroach first on diastasis (the slowest filling phase) so the effect on diastolic filling is minimized and cardiac output will increase. If other factors are held constant, the net effect of heart rate on cardiac output will depend mainly on the extent of rate increase, on atrial filling pressure and on the contractile or inotropic state of the ventricle.

If, at rest, the heart rate is progressively increased while atrial filling pressures remain normal, cardiac output will rise at first, then level off, and at rates of 120 to 130/min will begin to decline. However, during sympathoadrenal stimulation or exercise, cardiac output will only begin to decline at rates of about 180/min; this improved cardiac performance is due to a combination of increased venous return with increased atrial filling pressure and the inotropic effects mentioned above, i.e., increased strength of ventricular contraction and a shortening of ventricular systole (with a relative lengthening of diastole). This better performance is, however, contingent on the maintenance of adequate atrial filling pressure and volume; during exercise the increased metabolic rate, decrease in peripheral resistance especially in the exercising muscle and venoconstriction all contribute to the atrial filling so that the increase in heart rate will be associated with an increase in cardiac output in the young adult up to rates of about 180/min. With increasing age, this maximum rate will gradually decrease (Chapter 12).

Regulation of Heart Rate

While heart rate affects stroke volume as described above, it is a separately controlled variable which has other effects on cardiac performance. The chronotropic activity of the heart is normally determined by the rate of impulse generation in the SA node (Chapter 5). This, in turn, is influenced primarily by: (a) the autonomic balance between the sympathetic and vagal impulses to the node—sympathetic stimulation will increase heart rate and vagal stimulation will decrease it; (b) temperature and metabolic activity of the pacemaker tissue—increased temperature and metabolism will increase heart rate, reduced temperature and metabolism will have the reverse effect; and (c) influence on the heart of ionic and pH changes in the blood. The latter effects are less important from a heart rate standpoint.

ALTERATIONS IN CARDIAC OUTPUT

Physiological Alterations

A. *Exercise.* The greatest changes in cardiac output occur during intensive exercise with an increase in both rate and stroke volume; in this situation the cardiac output varies linearly with oxygen consumption and may be increased 4- to 6-fold (Chapter 12).

B. *Postural Changes.* On rising from a recumbent to an upright position the cardiac output decreases about 20% because of venous pooling in the lower extremities and a decrease in effective circulatory blood volume (Chapter 13).

C. *Pregnancy.* Cardiac output is increased partly because of increased body mass and partly because the blood vessels to the placenta and uterus may act as arteriovenous shunts to lower peripheral resistance; in the latter case cardiac output is then increased to maintain the blood pressure.

Pathological Alterations

These may be of several types:

A. *Blood Volume Changes.* In anemia, cardiac output is increased as a compensatory response to the circulatory hypoxia; in hemorrhagic and traumatic shock there is a pronounced decrease in cardiac output because of decreased blood volume.

B. *Metabolic Changes.* In fever and hyperthyroidism there is increased cardiac output due to increased metabolism and the relative circulatory hypoxia induced by the increased demand for oxygen.

C. *Peripheral Resistance Changes.* Opening of a large arteriovenous fistula will produce a sudden decrease in peripheral resistance and a rise in cardiac output.

D. *Heart Disease.* In early hypertension the elevated blood pressure is frequently associated with an increased cardiac output; later in the disease the hypertension is accompanied by an increased peripheral resistance (Chapter 15). In congestive heart failure, because of decreased cardiac contractility, there is reduced cardiac output and an inability to increase the output at ordinary work levels leading to shortness of breath and easy fatigability (Chapter 14).

MEASUREMENT OF CARDIAC OUTPUT

In experimental animals, cardiac output can be measured by placing an electromagnetic or ultrasonic flowmeter on the aorta or pulmonary artery for direct recording. In the human subject, the two most commonly used methods are the Fick and indicator-dilution methods. Both of these are "invasive" in the sense that they require cardiac catheterization for placement of a catheter into vessels close to the heart.

The Fick Method

In its passage through the lungs, the blood put out by the right ventricle takes up oxygen and gives up carbon dioxide. If the total oxygen consumption per unit time is determined with a respirometer, the increase of oxygen concentration in pulmonary venous blood will depend on the rate of blood flow, *i.e.*, right ventricular output per unit time. This, averaged over a period of time, is assumed to be equal to left ventricular output. The difference in oxygen content between mixed venous blood (from the pulmonary artery) and arterial blood represents the A − V oxygen difference. Then the cardiac output (CO) can be calculated:

$$CO = \frac{\text{Oxygen consumption (ml/min)}}{\text{A} - \text{Vo}_2 \text{ difference (ml/L)}}$$

Example

A resting subject with a heart rate of 80/min had an O_2 consumption of 250 ml/min. Blood samples taken simultaneously from the femoral artery by needle puncture and from the pulmonary artery through a cardiac catheter showed that his arterial blood contained 19.0 and his venous blood 15.0 ml O_2/100 ml blood. The arteriovenous oxygen difference was, therefore, 40 ml/L and cardiac output (CO) may be calculated as follows:

$$\frac{CO}{L/min} = \frac{250 \text{ ml/min}}{40 \text{ ml/L}}$$

$$= 6.25 \text{ L/min}$$

$$\text{Average stroke volume} = \frac{6,250 \text{ ml/min}}{80 \text{ beats/min}}$$

$$= 78 \text{ ml}$$

The Indicator-Dilution Method

This method involves the injection of a known amount of dye or other indicator substance into the circulation and the measurement of the dilution of this material during a known period of time. The indicator should be well mixed into the blood as it is injected, should not be lost from the circulation and must not be toxic or itself affect cardiac output.

Indocyanine green (cardiogreen), the dye most commonly used, satisfies most of these requirements. In practice a known amount of the dye is injected into the right heart *via* a cardiac catheter. A few seconds later the dye concentration is detected in arterial blood by withdrawing small samples of blood continuously from an arterial catheter and measuring the dye concentration with a photosensitive device called a densitometer.

The dye concentration gradually increases until it reaches a maximum and then it begins to decline until a second rise in concentration occurs as a result of recirculation. The downslope of the curve prior to recirculation approximates an exponential decay so that replotting the curve with the logarithm of dye concentration as the ordinate and time as the abscissa permits the time-concentration curve for the dye on its first circulation past the point of sampling to be defined by extrapolating the downslope. The inscribed curve will then indicate the average concentration of dye and the duration of this first passage. The volume of dye-containing blood that must have passed the sampling site per unit time in order to produce the curve can then be calculated by dividing the area of the curve into the amount of dye injected. It is evident that the larger the area under the curve, the smaller the cardiac output (Fig. 7-5).

Non-invasive Methods for Estimation of Cardiac Output and Performance

In the last several years there has been increasing emphasis in cardiovascular physiology on non-invasive methods. This has resulted not only from the higher cost and added risk of invasive techniques, but also because the emotional stress, which even minor invasive procedures sometimes invoke, produce their own physiological effects. Following are brief summaries of a few non-invasive techniques in current use.

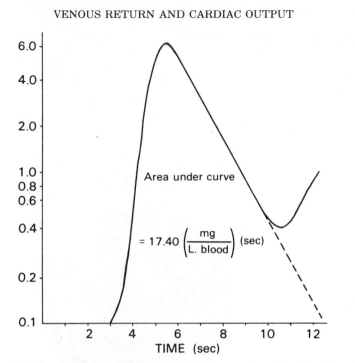

Figure 7-5. Curve of arterial indocyanine concentration after injection of 1.01 mg of dye into the pulmonary artery. Cardiac output = 1.01/17.40 = 0.058 L/ sec or 3.48 L/min. Ordinate indicates dye concentration in mg/L on a logarithmic scale.

A. Echocardiography. Reflected ultrasound is a widely used diagnostic technique in cardiology. High frequency sound waves from 2 to 3 megahertz are emitted and received by a transducer which is usually placed over the precordium. The wave pulses are reflected at interfaces between two media of different densities, amplified, displayed on an oscilloscope and recorded. A time-motion presentation displays moving structures as undulating lines. Echocardiography has proved particularly useful in visualization of valvular and pericardial abnormalities and recently for ventricular visualization (Fig. 7-6). From such data, estimates of EDV, ESV, SV and ejection fraction may be made.

B. Impedance Cardiography. The degree of distortion of an impedance wave from a high frequency current as transmitted through a moving column of fluid is proportional to the rate of flow of the fluid. Sensing of aortic flow in this manner by transthoracic impedance makes it possible to estimate cardiac output. Four thin, band electrodes

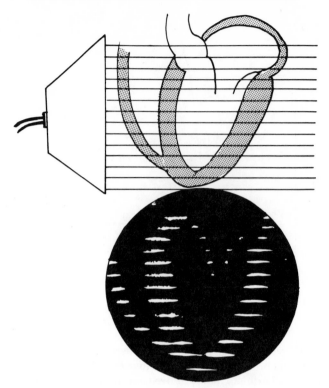

Figure 7-6. Two-dimensional echocardiographic image of ventricular walls developed from a linear array of ultrasonic transducer-receivers. (From R. F. Rushmer, *Cardiovascular Dynamics.* Philadelphia: W. B. Saunders Co., 1976.)

are usually placed about the neck and lower chest; the outer two electrodes are excited by a 100 kHz sinusoidal current and the resulting voltage monitored from the inner two electrodes. The waves are recorded with the impedance cardiograph and the relative stroke volume estimated with a formula developed by Kubicek and his colleagues (Fig. 7-7).

Cardiac output studies have shown good correlation between imped- ance and other standard methods and have indicated that impedance cardiography can provide a reliable index of relative changes in stroke volume.

C. Radionuclide Imaging. Another non-invasive method which has come into increasing use is the visualization of the cardiac chambers

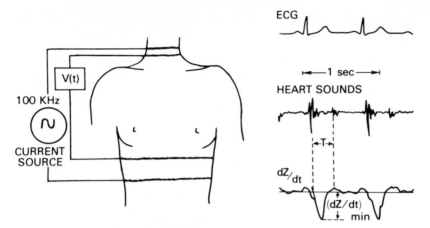

Figure 7-7. Transthoracic impedance cardiography. *Left,* rapid sinusoidal current is transmitted through the two outer electrodes and sensed by the inner ones. *Right,* the minimum value of the first derivative of the main impedance wave (dZ/dt min) and the ventricular ejection time (T) are used to calculate the stroke volume.

with radioisotopes. The intravenous injection of a small bolus of a gamma emitter such as ^{99m}Tc pertechnetate permits rapid sequential visualization of the heart, great vessels and pulmonary vasculature by use of an Anger scintillation camera; the image is usually recorded and stored on tape. EDV and ejection fraction may be determined; the recent development of portable bedside units has increased the clinical practicality of this technique. Radionuclide imaging appears to have considerable potential and will undoubtedly come into increasing use.

REFERENCES

FEIGENBAUM, H.: *Echocardiography.* Philadelphia: Lea & Febiger, 1972.

FOLKOW, B., AND E. NEIL: *Circulation.* New York: Oxford University Press, 1971.

GUYTON, A. C.: *Circulatory Physiology: Cardiac Output and Its Regulation.* Philadelphia: W. B. Saunders Co., 1973.

KUBICEK, W. G., F. J. KOTTKE, M. U. RAMOS, R. P. PATTERSON, D. A. WITTSOE, J. W. LABREE, W. REMOLE, T. E. LAYMAN, H. SCHOENING, AND J. T. GARAMELLA: The Minnesota impedance cardiograph—theory and application. *Biomed. Eng.* 9:410–416, 1974.

RUSHMER, R. F.: *Cardiovascular Dynamics.* Philadelphia: W. B. Saunders Co., 1976.

SMITH, J. J., J. E. BUSH, V. T. WIEDMEIER, AND F. E. TRISTANI: Application of impedance cardiography to study of postural stress. *J. Appl. Physiol.* 29: 133, 1970.

SCHER, A.: Control of cardiac output. In *Physiology and Biophysics*, ed. by T. C. Ruch and H. D. Patton. Philadelphia: W. B. Saunders Co., 1974.

STRAUSS, H. W., B. PITT, AND A. E. JAMES: *Cardiovascular Nuclear Medicine.* St. Louis: C. V. Mosby Co., 1974.

chapter 8

The Microcirculation and the Lymphatic System

ANATOMY OF THE MICROCIRCULATION

That portion of the systemic and pulmonary circulation especially adapted for exchange of water, gases, nutrients and waste material is known as the microcirculation. It is, in a sense, the most important part of the cardiovascular system since it is here that its ultimate objective, *i.e.*, the exchange with tissue cells, is realized. While the microcirculation is considered a closed system, its walls are much more permeable than those of any other part of the circulation.

As shown in Figure 8-1, microcirculatory vessels have an irregular course and configuration; because of their great cross-sectional area, the flow velocity is least at this point. This slowing of the stream and dispersal over a maximum surface makes the microcirculation particularly suitable for exchange. It has been estimated that because of the enormous number and wide distribution of capillaries, individual cells are seldom more than 40 to 80 μm from a capillary surface. Arterioles

129

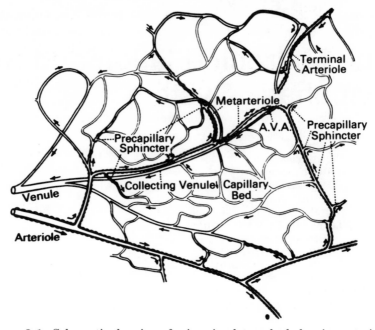

Figure 8-1. Schematic drawing of microcirculatory bed showing arterioles, metarterioles, capillaries and venules. Note precapillary sphincters at points where capillaries branch off from the metarterioles. (From B. W. Zweifach, *Conference on High Blood Pressure.* New York: Macy Foundation, 1950.)

are highly muscular vessels but metarterioles, which generally come off the arterioles at right angles, have only a single discontinuous smooth muscle layer in their walls.

The metarterioles serve to some extent as through-channels to the venules, which are much larger and have a greater capacity than the arterioles. At the point where capillaries branch off the metarterioles, a thin band of muscle, *i.e.*, the precapillary sphincter, encircles the capillary; these sphincters serve as the main control over capillary flow.

CAPILLARIES

Capillaries of different tissues vary considerably, both anatomically and functionally. These differences are usually related to the special role of the respective tissue or organ and will be discussed further in

Chapter 11 (Circulation to Special Regions). In the skin, for example, particularly of the toes, fingers and ears, there are arteriovenous anastomoses (AVAs) which are wide-bore, direct channels between the arterioles and venules. Unlike capillaries of other organs, the AVAs are under neurogenic control; their shunting capabilities enable them to reduce heat loss through the skin during cold exposure.

The true capillaries are the most important functional units of the microcirculation. They are short, narrow tubes, about 7 to 10 μm in diameter with a wall consisting of a single layer of endothelial cells and a basement membrane; they have no smooth muscle (Fig. 8-2). Between adjacent endothelial cells are slit-like pores or clefts which range from about 50 to 90 Å in width but which are frequently constricted at one point to about 40 Å.

The cytoplasm of the endothelial cells usually contains pinocytotic vesicles which are believed to play a role in transport processes across the cell. Although there are a wide variety of capillary structures among the different tissues, three main types have been distinguished by electron microscopy on the basis of the continuity of their filtration

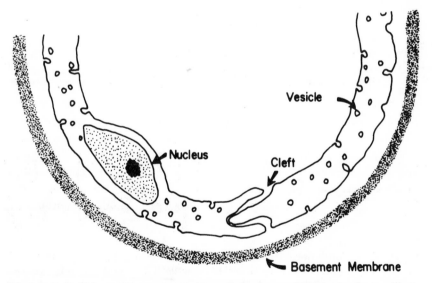

Figure 8-2. Schematic representation of electron micrograph of a capillary. Note the slit-pore (cleft) between the endothelial cells. (From C. A. Wiederhielm, in *Physiology and Biophysics*, ed. by T. C. Ruch and H. D. Patton. Philadelphia: W. B. Saunders Co., 1974.)

barriers; these have been labelled continuous, fenestrated and discontinuous types.

Continuous Capillaries

These are capillaries with no recognizable intercellular openings; one sub-group with a "low" or flattened cellular type is seen mainly in muscle, nerve and adipose tissue; a second sub-group with a "high" or cuboidal epithelial structure is more common in lymph nodes and the thymus gland (Fig. 8-3, *upper*).

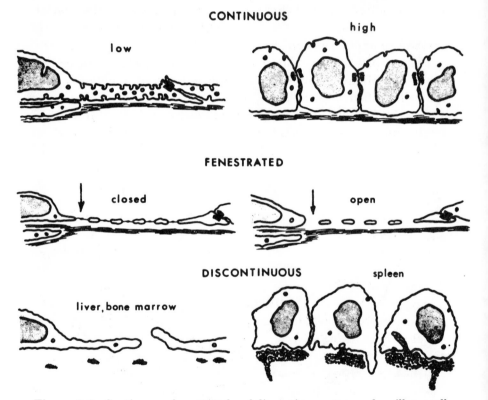

Figure 8-3. Continuous, fenestrated and discontinuous types of capillary wall as shown by schematics of electron micrographs. The classification is based on the completeness of the endothelial layer and in general parallels the extent of the physical barrier to filtration. (From G. Majno, in *Handbook of Physiology*, Section 2: *Circulation*, vol. III, ed. by W. F. Hamilton and P. Dow. Washington, D.C.: American Physiological Society, 1965.)

Fenestrated Capillaries

This type of capillary (Fig. 8-3, *middle*) has small gaps which are either "closed" as in endocrine glands and intestinal villi or "open" as in renal glomeruli. These gaps usually range from 800 to 1000 Å and are, therefore, about 15 to 20 times wider than those of the continuous capillaries.

Discontinuous Capillaries

This type of membrane (Fig. 8-3, *lower*) has an endothelium with large intercellular gaps; these vessels are usually referred to as sinusoids and are typical of liver, bone marrow and spleen. It should be pointed out that the so-called "tight" junctions of the continuous capillaries are sufficiently wide to permit rapid diffusion of small molecular substances. There is no barrier to diffusion of gases. The other two types of capillaries with larger gaps have much greater permeability, so that in the sinusoids, large proteins and even cells can pass. Thus, to a large extent the transfer of substances between the capillaries and interstitial fluid can be correlated with these anatomical differences in capillary structure.

REGULATION OF THE MICROCIRCULATION

As mentioned in Chapter 1, the mean intravascular pressures in the capillary range from about 25 to 30 mm Hg at the arteriolar end to about 8 to 10 mm Hg at the venular end. Flow through the arterioles and metarterioles is controlled mainly by the sympathetic vasoconstrictors on the basis of circulatory reflexes as will be described in Chapters 9 and 10. Flow through the capillaries, however, is not under neural control; rather it is regulated by the precapillary sphincters which are, in turn, influenced by the local metabolic state of the tissue—a process called autoregulation (Chapter 9).

Thus, flow through individual capillary areas can be adjusted to meet both the local demands of the tissues and the overall control of the circulation. Rate of flow through individual capillary beds can vary considerably. In skeletal muscle, for example, only about 5 to 10% of the capillaries are open at rest; with increased metabolic activity, the precapillary sphincters open widely, probably in response to the accumulation of metabolites. As flow is restored and O_2 needs are satisfied, the sphincters again close. Because of the large number of capillaries, some open, some closed, regional flow will reflect the average value through the entire bed.

TRANSCAPILLARY EXCHANGE

Movement across the capillary wall is influenced by several factors, *i.e.*, (a) the type and molecular size of the substance being transported, (b) the balance of hydrostatic and colloid osmotic forces across the membrane, (c) the capillary surface available for exchange, and (d) the physical characteristics of the capillary membrane.

The continuous type of capillary is found most often in muscle, connective tissue, the pulmonary circulation and brain. Consequently the filtration coefficient (*i.e.*, the rate of filtration per unit pressure difference) is relatively low in these tissues. In the renal glomerulus and intestinal mucosa, which have fenestrated capillaries, the filtration rate is moderate to high. In the hepatic sinusoids and spleen with discontinuous or practically "open" capillaries, molecules of all sizes pass readily; these tissues "leak" the greatest amounts of protein and have the highest interstitial plasma protein concentrations.

There are two general methods—*viz.* diffusion and filtration—by which substances pass through capillary walls, depending mainly on their lipid solubility. These are discussed in the following sections.

Diffusion

This is the most important transcapillary exchange mechanism and may take place through the intercellular slit-like pores or through the cell wall itself. Lipid-soluble materials such as oxygen, carbon dioxide and certain anesthetic agents diffuse rapidly with little hindrance through the lipoprotein membrane of the endothelial cell wall. Water-soluble substances on the other hand are limited to diffusion through the intercellular slit-pores in which case the molecular movement is aided by the physical process of filtration.

Filtration-Absorption

Starling described the exchange of fluid across the capillary wall on the basis of the hydrostatic and osmotic pressures on each side of the membrane (law of the capillary). Later, Landis provided specific pressure measurements to verify this concept; Landis found hydrostatic pressures of about 32 and 15 mm Hg in the arteriolar and venular end of a capillary respectively and plasma osmotic pressures due to plasma proteins (oncotic pressures) of about 25 mm Hg. According to the Starling-Landis concept, there is, as a consequence, a resultant pressure gradient along the capillary which governs transport across the capillary wall (Fig. 8-4).

At the arterial end, there is an excess of hydrostatic over osmotic pressure tending to promote filtration (movement into the tissue) and at the venous end an excess of osmotic over hydrostatic pressure tending to promote reabsorption. In the intermediate region there is a gradual decline in filtration and a beginning of reabsorption. It will be

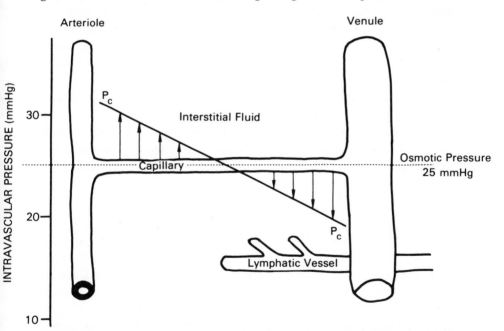

Figure 8-4. Schematic diagram showing filtration and reabsorption along an average capillary. P_c is the capillary hydrostatic pressure, which decreases progressively from the arteriolar to the venular side. The relation of P_c to capillary osmotic pressure causes filtration on the arteriolar side and reabsorption on the venular side. (Adapted from E. M. Landis and J. R. Pappenheimer, in *Handbook of Physiology*, Section 2: *Circulation*, vol. II, ed. by W. F. Hamilton and P. Dow. Washington, D.C.: American Physiological Society, 1963.)

noticed that the areas under the triangles are approximately equal, indicating that filtration and absorption are also balanced and about equal. Further studies have indicated that the total amount of water filtered through the capillaries of the body is about 20 liters per day; of this amount, about 16 to 18 liters are reabsorbed into the capillaries; the remaining 2 to 4 liters per day are removed by the lymphatic system and returned to the circulation.

Although Figure 8-4 refers only to capillary hydrostatic (P_c) and plasma oncotic (π_p) pressures, the interstitial hydrostatic (P_i) and interstitial osmotic pressures (π_i) must also be considered. While P_i and π_i are both quite low compared to the respective P_c and π_p values, the interstitial pressures may, in pathological circumstances, increase and become significant factors in transcapillary fluid exchange as described later in this chapter. Therefore, a more accurate definition of transcapillary forces would be the balance between the net trans-mural hydrostatic pressure (P_c-P_i) and the net transmural oncotic pressure (π_p-π_i).

Two thirds or more of the oncotic effect of the 7 g/dl of plasma proteins is due to albumin. Because of their large molecular size only a small percentage of plasma protein diffuses across the capillary wall in most tissues. However, as previously mentioned, in the sinusoids, the plasma proteins move more easily into the interstitial fluid so that π_i begins to approach π_p.

CAPILLARY PERMEABILITY

As previously stated, the transport of material across the capillary wall depends not only on diffusion and on the balance of pressures across the capillary but also on the structure and porosity of the wall and the nature of the material being transported. For water-soluble substances which are transported primarily *via* the slit-pores, a single mathematical expression can be used to describe the movement across the capillary wall, *i.e.*:

$$F = (P)(S)[(P_c\text{-}P_i) - (\pi_p\text{-}\pi_i)]$$

in which F is the net movement of fluid, P is the specific permeability of the capillary and S is the capillary surface area perfused—which depends mainly on the number of capillaries open to flow. P_c and P_i are the hydrostatic pressures in the capillary and interstitial fluid, and

π_p and π_i are the osmotic pressure values in the plasma and interstitial fluid respectively. The right side of the equation is a restatement of the balance of hydrostatic and osmotic forces previously described; as will be noted, if F is positive there will be an outward transport of fluid from the capillary and if negative an inward one.

In Table 8-1 are listed the specific permeabilities of a few common substances as well as their molecular weights and sizes. As will be noted in the continuous or tight capillary which prevails in muscle, the permeability ranges from high values for the smaller molecules to practical impermeability for the larger protein molecules; this is consistent with the concept that the movement of these substances across the capillary barrier is essentially a passive one dependent mainly on physical forces. The permeability factor may be affected by hypoxia, drugs and certain pathological conditions.

LYMPHATIC SYSTEM

The lymphatics comprise a type of secondary interstitial drainage system supplementing venular drainage. Lymphatics are porous, thin-walled vessels resembling capillaries. From closed, blind ends lying in the interstitial space, lymph channels drain centrally and are occasionally interrupted by lymph nodes; inside the nodes the vessels break up into numerous sinuses, lined by lymphoid cells, which reunite into

Table 8-1. Permeability of Mammalian Muscle Capillaries to Some Water-Soluble Molecules

Substance	Molecular Weight	Approximate Molecular Radius (Å)	Specific Permeability*
H_2O	18	1.5	28
NaCl	58	2.3	15
Urea	60	2.6	14
Glucose	180	3.7	6
Sucrose	342	4.8	4
Inulin	5,500	12–15	0.3
Myoglobin	17,000	19	0.1
Serum albumin	67,000	36	0.001

* Expressed as mol/sec/cm^2 of membrane per mol/concentration difference $\times$ 10^5. (From E. M. Landis and J. R. Pappenheimer, in *Handbook of Physiology*, Section 2: *Circulation*, vol. II, ed. by W. F. Hamilton and P. Dow. Washington, D.C.: American Physiological Society, 1963.)

efferent lymph channels. Ultimately, all the lymphatics empty into two main trunks, the thoracic duct (on the left) and the right lymphatic duct; these drain into the junctions of the subclavian and internal jugular veins on their respective sides. The primary function of the lymphatic system is to clear the interstitial spaces of excess fluid, protein, lipids and foreign materials.

Lymph resembles interstitial tissue fluid with which it is in close equilibrium; its composition is similar to plasma except that its average protein concentration is lower, i.e., about 2 g/dl. The highest protein concentration is that of hepatic lymph which has a range of about 5 to 6 g/dl. Pressure in the lymphatics has generally been believed to be similar to that of interstitial fluid, i.e., about 1 to 2 mm Hg. Guyton and his colleagues have reported that interstitial pressure normally is about −6 mm Hg; these investigators believe that this negative pressure is important to maintain the tissue spaces relatively dry so that diffusion distances between capillaries and cells are optimally short.

Lymph flow is relatively sluggish and total flow in man is about 2 to 4 L/day. This flow is increased by muscular activity or massage, increased venous pressure, hyperemia or inflammation. Lymphatic vessels are highly permeable and are capable of picking up large particles, e.g., dying blood cells, carbon, bacteria, and foreign particles. Intestinal lymphatics (lacteals) pick up large lipid globules, i.e., chylomicra after a fat meal.

EDEMA

Edema is the accumulation of excess fluid in the interstitial spaces of the body. Clinical edema usually develops in dependent areas such as the feet and becomes more evident in tissues in which expansion is limited, e.g., around the eyes. Edema may be produced in several ways as described in the following:

General Increase in Venous Pressure

As is shown in Figure 8-4 and also in Figure 8-5A, if there is a normal balance of filtration and reabsorption forces, there will be no accumulation of interstitial fluid. However, if the pressure is consistently increased in the veins, it will also rise in the venules and eventually in the arterial end of the capillary; this will result in an increase in

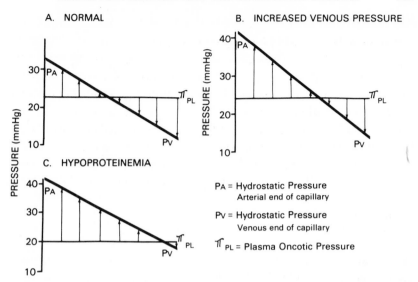

Figure 8-5. Effect of variations in hydrostatic and colloid osmotic pressures on fluid filtration—reabsorption balance. *A.* Normal balance of capillary hydrostatic and plasma oncotic pressures. *B.* Elevation of venular and capillary pressure with excessive filtration and increased interstitial fluid. *C.* Decreased plasma protein and plasma oncotic pressure, with excessive capillary filtration and tendency toward edema.

filtration and in the accumulation of interstitial fluid illustrated by the net force tending to move fluid out of the capillary (Fig. 8-5*B*). This occurs most commonly in congestive heart failure with elevation of right ventricular end-diastolic pressure, venous congestion and a resultant dependent edema (discussed further in Chapter 14).

Hypoproteinemia

If the plasma protein decreases to a low level, the plasma oncotic pressure will also fall so that the capillary hydrostatic pressure overbalances the oncotic pressure with a tendency for fluid accumulation in the tissue spaces. The loss of plasma protein—primarily albumin—occurs most commonly in nephrosis, in which large amounts of albumin are continuously lost in the urine, in nutritional edema in which there is inadequate protein in the diet and with severe burns in which the capillaries are damaged.

Lymphatic Obstruction

If the small amount of protein that continually "leaks" through the capillary walls and is normally returned *via* the lymph, cannot be reabsorbed, it will accumulate in the tissue until it reaches a significant concentration and prevents the return of fluid into the venular end of the capillary. This occurs rarely but when seen is usually due to a tropical parasitic disease called "Filariasis"; the larvae (microfilaria) gradually obstruct the lymphatic vessels. The edema may become so excessive that a leg may swell to two or three times its normal size— hence the clinical term "elephantiasis" for this type of massive edema.

Local Edema

Localized edema may occur in an organ or region if there is extensive venous obstruction with elevation of venous and capillary pressures, *e.g.*, a widespread venous thrombosis.

REFERENCES

GUYTON, A. C., H. J. GRANGER, AND A. E. TAYLOR: Interstitial fluid pressure. *Physiol. Rev.* 51:527, 1971.

HADDY, F. J., J. B. SCOTT, AND G. J. GREGA: Peripheral circulation: fluid transfer across the microvascular membrane. In *Cardiovascular Physiology II*, vol. 9, International Review of Physiology, ed. by A. C. Guyton, Baltimore: University Park Press, 1976.

INTAGLIETTA, M., AND P. C. JOHNSON: *Principles of Capillary Exchange in Peripheral Circulation*, ed. by P. C. Johnson. New York: John Wiley & Sons, 1978.

LANDIS, E. M., AND J. R. PAPPENHEIMER: Exchange of substances through the capillary walls. In *Handbook of Physiology*, Section 2: *Circulation*, vol. II, ed. by W. F. Hamilton and P. Dow. Washington, D.C.: American Physiological Society, 1963.

MAJNO, G.: Ultrastructure of vascular membrane. In *Handbook of Physiology*, Section 2: *Circulation*, vol. III, ed. by W. F. Hamilton and P. Dow. Washington, D.C.: American Physiological Society, 1965.

NICOLL, P. A., AND A. E. TAYLOR: Lymph formation and flow. *Annu. Rev. Physiol.* 39:73–95, 1977.

RENKIN, E. M.: Multiple pathways of capillary permeability. *Circ. Res.* 41: 735–742, 1977.

WIEDERHIELM, C. A.: Dynamics of transcapillary fluid exchange. *J. Gen. Physiol.* 52:29–63, 1968.

chapter 9

The Peripheral Circulation and Its Regulation

NORMAL DISTRIBUTION OF BLOOD FLOW

How blood flow is distributed to the various organs is obviously of considerable importance; total flow is limited and it must be disposed only in amounts needed when and where it is needed. If, in a 70-kg adult, a cardiac output of 5400 ml/min were partitioned evenly on a weight basis, the mean flow would be about 7.7 ml/min/100 g of tissue. However, the actual distribution is quite uneven. Figure 9-1 shows average values for tissue blood flow and oxygen consumption in the normal adult human at rest.

As the top bar graph shows, three tissues, liver (hepatosplanchnic region), kidney and skeletal muscle receive about two thirds of the total flow. If the organ flows are divided by the respective organ weights, the blood flow per unit weight or "vascularity" (Fig. 9-1, 3rd graph) is obtained. As described in Chapter 2, when comparing relative

141

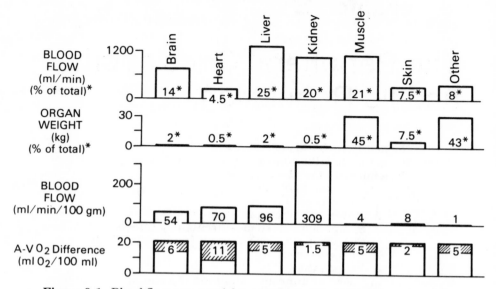

Figure 9-1. Blood flow, organ weight, vascularity (blood flow per unit weight) and A-V oxygen extraction of main organs in normal adult at rest. Body weight, 70 kg; cardiac output, 5400 ml/min; mean vascularity, 7.7 ml/min/100 g; mean A-V O_2 difference, 5 ml O_2 per dl. (Liver flow includes that of the intestinal and other organs draining into the portal vein and therefore actually refers to hepatosplanchnic flow.)

flow or peripheral resistance values, it is necessary to consider the weight of the respective organ or organism.

Four organs, *viz.*, kidney, liver, heart and brain all have a high flow/ unit weight because of a relatively low vascular resistance/unit weight; in contrast *resting* skeletal muscle and the relatively avascular tissues such as skin, bone, cartilage, fat and connective tissue *etc.*, which are grouped under "other," have a low blood flow/unit weight because of their relatively high vascular resistance.

The kidneys, being primarily clearance organs, obviously need a very large flow to carry out their function; their close proximity through short arterial vessels to the high aortic pressure and their innate vascularity contribute to the high resting flow. The renal clearance function is associated with only a modest oxygen demand so that the flow is mainly "non-nutritional." As a consequence, the renal A-V oxygen difference is small, *i.e.*, 1.5 ml of O_2/100 ml of blood. Therefore, in spite of the very large flow, the estimated oxygen consumption of the kidneys, *i.e.*, about 4.6 ml/min/100 g (3.09 × 1.5), is less than that of the liver (4.8) or heart (7.7) (Fig. 9-1).

That fraction of the arterial O_2 content taken up in the tissues is usually termed the O_2 extraction ratio. If the arterial O_2 content were 20 ml/dl, the O_2 extraction for resting skeletal muscle (Fig. 9-1) would be 0.25 and for myocardium 0.55. The remaining fraction of unextracted oxygen represents an important reserve.

In certain stress situations, both the total flow and flow distribution shown in Figure 9-1 (*top graph*) would be considerably altered. For example, during severe exercise, cardiac output can increase 4 to 6 times; furthermore, the percentage of total flow received by skeletal muscle would increase to about 90% because of a marked decrease in vascular resistance in the dilated muscle vessels (Chapter 12). Since, in addition to the increased fractional flow to muscle, there will also be an increase in the O_2 extraction ratio in muscle tissue, the total O_2 consumption of skeletal muscle can, in severe exercise, increase 15 to 20 times over the resting level.

RANGE OF FLOW RESPONSES IN DIFFERENT ORGANS

Changes in vessel caliber may occur passively as the transmural pressure changes or through active contraction (vasoconstriction) or relaxation (vasodilation) of its circular smooth muscle; such activity will, in the small arteries and arterioles, mainly influence peripheral resistance, but in the small veins and venules, the primary effect is on the capacitance of the peripheral bed.

Vessel caliber may change over a wide range; vasoconstriction of small arterial vessels may be so intense that flow practically ceases; on the other hand if all constrictor nerves are cut and the vessels maximally dilated by pharmacological agents, flow may increase 2- or 3-fold in the brain and liver, 5-fold in the myocardium and over 20-fold in skeletal muscle (Fig. 9-2). In contrast to this, renal vessels can only increase their flow about 16%. Such large flow alterations are possible because of the fourth power effect of the radius on flow (Chapter 2).

PRINCIPLES OF FLOW REGULATION

Given its inherent vascular architecture, altered flow demands might be met either by a change in the central perfusion pressure or by

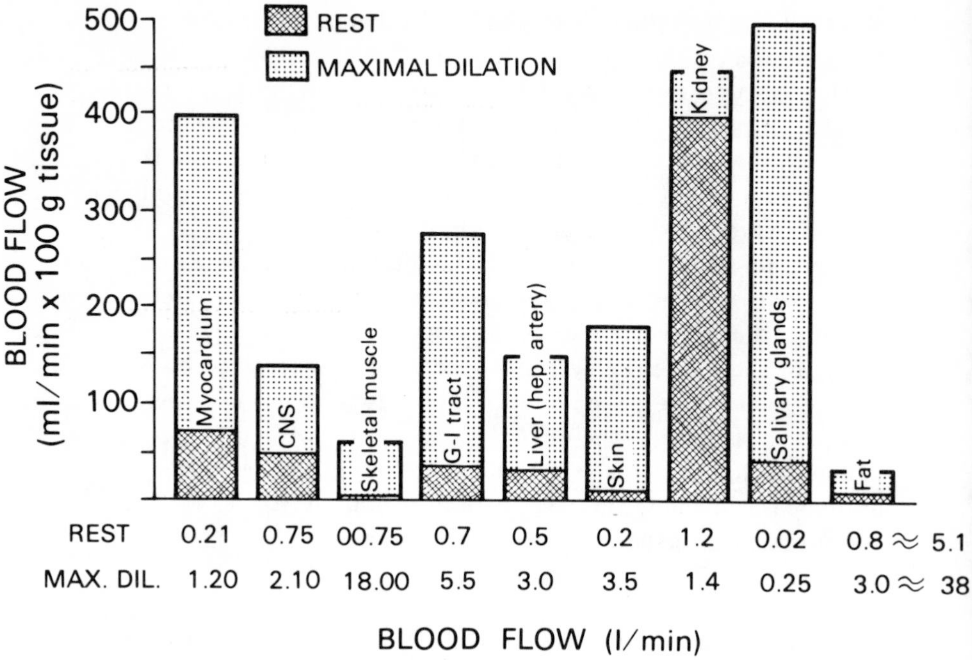
REST
MAXIMAL DILATION
BLOOD FLOW
(ml/min x 100 g tissue)
500
400
300
200
100
Myocardium
CNS
Skeletal muscle
G-I tract
Liver (hep. artery)
Skin
Kidney
Salivary glands
Fat
REST 0.21 0.75 00.75 0.7 0.5 0.2 1.2 0.02 0.8 ≈ 5.1
MAX. DIL. 1.20 2.10 18.00 5.5 3.0 3.5 1.4 0.25 3.0 ≈ 38
BLOOD FLOW (l/min)

Figure 9-2. Regional blood flow at rest (*shaded areas*) and at maximal dilation (*stippled areas*) per organ and per 100 g tissue. (From S. Mellander and B. Johansson, *Pharmacol. Rev.* 20:117, 1968.)

adjustment of vessel caliber. From an organism standpoint, it is most efficient to maintain arterial pressure relatively constant in order to insure adequate coronary and cerebral flow and to meet the peripheral demands through adjustment of individual resistances. In effect this is what normally occurs; the primary objective of this chapter is to consider how this is brought about. The adjustment of vessel caliber is accomplished by two general mechanisms i.e. through central regulation and local regulation.

A. Central Regulation of Flow

This refers either to *neural control*, done almost entirely by the sympathetic nervous system, or to *humoral control*, which refers to the effects of catecholamines or other blood-borne agents such as O_2, CO_2, Ca^{++}, K^+ or H^+ ions. Both of these regulating factors are "central," *i.e.*, they originate from a source remote from the tissue affected.

B. Local Regulation of Flow

This is carried out by metabolites, O_2, CO_2, "local hormones" or various ions, which are derived in the individual tissues and act directly on the nearby capillary beds.

In considering the regulation of blood flow to an organ or organism, an important distinction must be made between short- and long-term circulatory adjustments, *i.e.*, those made rapidly over minutes or hours in contrast to those which occur over days and weeks. The mechanisms involved in these two processes are quite different. In the following sections, the short-term adaptations will be considered first and in greater detail.

In the final section of the chapter, long-term regulation of flow will be discussed in general; in succeeding chapters vascular luminal adjustments of greater duration which apply to specific situations will be described at some length. These will include circulatory changes which develop during physical training and those incident to aging (Chapter 12) and circulatory adjustments which occur in pathological circumstances such as Ischemic Heart Disease (Chapter 14), Congestive Heart Failure (Chapter 14) and Hypertension (Chapter 15).

CENTRAL REGULATION OF FLOW

Neural Control of Flow

A. Autonomic Transmitters and Receptors

The autonomic nervous system (ANS), which includes the thoracolumbar (sympathetic) outflow and the craniosacral (parasympathetic) outflow, is responsible for integrating and modulating the functions of all the autonomous organs of the body, including the cardiovascular system. Neural transmission along the ANS is done in the usual fashion, *i.e.*, by means of self-propagating action potentials; transmission across synapses and across junctions with other tissues is *via* rather unique and specific chemical agents known as neurohumoral transmitters. These transmitters combine with receptors on the effector cells to activate the end-organ.

Basically there are three transmitters involved in the ANS: (a) *acetylcholine* (ACh), released at all "cholinergic" endings, *i.e.*, at ANS ganglia, at parasympathetic endings and at voluntary nerve muscle junctions; (b) *norepinephrine* (NE) released at all sympathetic "adrenergic" endings; and (c) *epinephrine*, liberated (along with a small fraction of NE) by the adrenal medulla into the blood.

If the transmitter agent (*e.g.*, NE or ACh) is injected so that it reaches the receptors *via* the blood stream, the humoral effect will be similar to the neural one so that a "sympathomimetic" or "parasympathomimetic" effect will be produced. But whether generated by neural or humoral means, autonomic effects on the various end-organs are diverse and complex. A significant (and initially baffling) discovery was that specific chemicals could prevent or competitively "block" certain autonomic effects (but not others) and thus render the transmitter temporarily ineffective at these sites.

In 1948, Ahlquist proposed that these divergent sympathetic responses were due to the existence of two different types of "receptors" at the various anatomical sites, which responded differently to the transmitters. These he called "alpha" and "beta" receptors. Because NE, either by neural or humoral route, will produce a strong vasoconstriction of the blood vessels of skin, kidney, splanchnic area and skeletal muscle (*i.e.*, a "pure" vasoconstriction), he assumed that such receptors were abundant at these sites. At other sites, *e.g.*, in vessels of the brain and heart, NE will produce limited or no constriction since at these locations such receptors are scarce. These were called alpha receptors and the action an alpha constrictor action. Alpha receptors are activated by NE and less strongly by E.

Specific agents such as phenoxybenzamine (Dibenzyline) or phentolamine (Regitine) will block alpha (but not beta) receptors and thus—depending on the dose—will minimize or prevent the alpha vasoconstriction. The rapid and effective increase in peripheral vascular resistance produced by reflex sympathetic alpha constriction is an important defense mechanism against a blood pressure fall, *e.g.*, during hemorrhage. An animal previously injected with a strong alpha blocking dose of phenoxybenzamine will have a much lesser resistance to hemorrhage than a control animal.

Beta receptors are most prevalent in the heart and in blood vessels of skeletal muscle and are activated by epinephrine or by one of its analogues, isoproterenol (Isoprel). When occupied by the transmitter, beta receptors initiate (a) increased heart rate and contractile strength of the myocardium and (b) a "pure" vasodilation of skeletal muscle blood vessels. Beta receptors (but not alpha) can be blocked by diisoproterenol (Propranolol). Propranolol is used in the treatment of certain types of hypertension and can assist in controlling blood pressure by reducing inotropic activity of the ventricle.

There is a third type of postganglionic sympathetic nerve ending, *i.e.*, cholinergic, located only in vessels of skeletal muscle; these endings, rather paradoxically, release ACh which stimulates "cholinergic" (or more specifically "muscarinic") receptors and causes vasodilation. This effect, which can be blocked by the primary muscarinic blocking agent, atropine, is thought to be involved in certain emotional responses such as fright or rage.

Parasympathetic control of blood flow (to be discussed later in this chapter) is much more limited than that of the sympathetic system.

The synthesis of catecholamines is outlined in a simplified diagram in Figure 9-3. NE, derived in a series of steps from tyrosine, is for the most part, synthesized locally by the adrenergic nerve cell. About 80% is removed *via* reuptake into the neuron or by diffusion into surrounding fluids or blood. Most of the remainder is metabolically degraded. The importance of the uptake process lies in the consequent availability (or not) of the NE for continued combination with the effector and so is a determinant of the strength and duration of the NE effect. The NE secreted by the nerve cell remains active for only a few seconds but that secreted by the adrenal medulla can remain active for several minutes.

Aside from alpha, beta and cholinergic receptors, recent investigations have indicated the likelihood of "dopaminergic" receptors. Dopamine, which is only one of the intermediate compounds in the synthetic pathway of NE, has a vasodilator effect on renal and splanchnic vascular beds, which action can be blocked by other specific agents.

It has been shown that in congestive heart failure, there is a depletion of myocardial catecholamines, with consequent reduction of inotropic capability. The depletion is probably due to a marked reduction of tyrosine hydroxylase, the rate-limiting enzyme in the conversion of tyrosine to DOPA.

As is evident from the above, certain tissues, by virtue of having different kinds of receptors, are capable of different types of vascular response if the proper stimuli are provided. This is particularly true of skeletal muscle. Figure 9-4 illustrates the effects of successive blockade

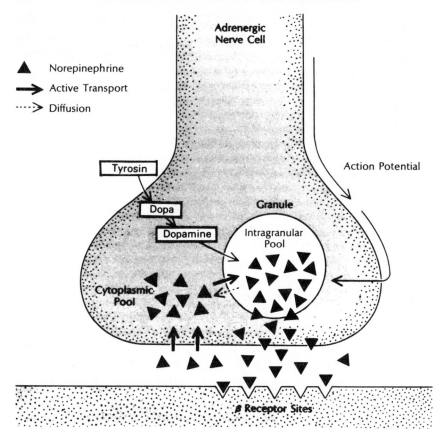

Figure 9-3. Schema showing local synthesis and release of norepinephrine (NE) in the heart. Ninety per cent of the cardiac NE is synthesized locally. The NE is stored, either in the granules or in the cytoplasm, and is released by the action potential. It then leaves the nerve cell, attaches to the myocardial beta receptor site and stimulates myocardial contraction. (From E. Braunwald, *The Myocardium: Failure and Infarction.* New York: HP Publishing Co., 1974.)

of different receptors on skeletal muscle blood flow. Skeletal muscle, because it comprises about 45% of the body bulk and has unusual constrictor and dilator capabilities, represents an enormous pool of vascular resistance.

B. The Sympathetic System—Circulatory Effects

Descending fibers from the cardiac and vasomotor centers of the medulla synapse with cells of the intermediolateral cell column of the

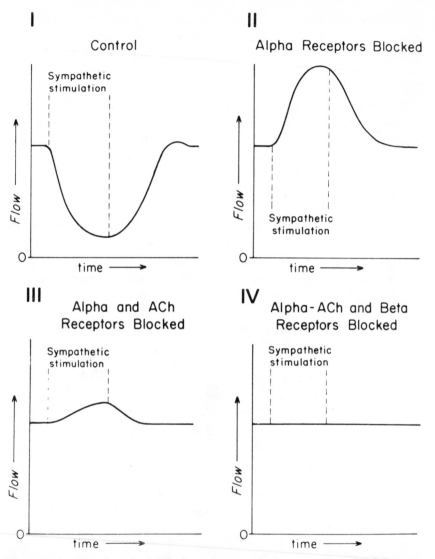

Figure 9-4. Results of stimulation of sympathetic nerves on blood flow in skeletal muscle. *I,* a strong vasoconstriction is present due to alpha receptor action; *II,* after alpha blockade, a sympathetic vasodilator effect is unmasked; *III,* after atropine the main vasodilator action in *II* is shown to be due to sympathetic cholinergic action. In *IV* the smaller, residual vasodilator action (beta effect) is abolished with a beta blocker. (From T. C. Ruch and H. D. Patton, *Physiology and Biophysics.* Philadelphia: W. B. Saunders Co., 1974.)

spinal cord; preganglionic fibers from the cord travel *via* the anterior spinal roots to the thoracolumbar sympathetic chain (Fig. 9-5). Descending impulses from the cerebral cortex and hypothalamus may also, by way of these spinal pathways, induce sympathetic vascular responses.

Postganglionic fibers from the cervical and upper four thoracic sympathetic ganglia supply the heart (SA and AV nodes and myocardium). Stimulation of these fibers activate beta adrenergic receptors and cause increase in rate and conduction velocity in the heart (Chapter 5) and increased myocardial contractility (Chapter 6).

Other sympathetic postganglionic fibers join the somatic and other autonomic nerves to reach practically all arteries and veins of the body. Upon stimulation, these fibers activate alpha adrenergic receptors to produce a general vasoconstriction, particularly marked in the skin, skeletal muscle, splanchnic and renal vascular beds. Sympathetic stimulation will also activate peripheral beta adrenergic receptors which will tend to produce vasodilation, particularly in skeletal muscle;

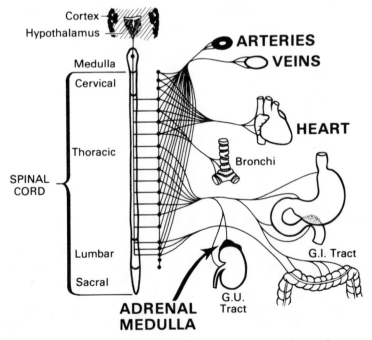

Figure 9-5. Sympathetic pathways to the heart and vasculature.

however, as previously mentioned, this vasodilator tendency in the muscle is masked by the stronger alpha constrictor action.

Preganglionic sympathetic fibers supply the adrenal medulla where they control the release of adrenal catecholamines into the blood stream.

Sympathetic stimulation will produce other important, non-circulatory effects, *e.g.*, relaxation of smooth muscle of the respiratory bronchioles, gastrointestinal tract and urinary tract and lessened secretion of sweat and lacrimal glands. Sympathetic stimulation also increases hepatic and muscle glycogenolysis and induces hyperglycemia; these metabolic effects assist in energy maintenance during prolonged stress such as physical exercise.

C. Parasympathetic System—Circulatory Effects

Preganglionic fibers of the craniosacral division of ANS arise either in motor nuclei of the brain stem, and exit with the cranial nerves, or in the sacral division of the spinal cord (Fig. 9-6).

The vagus (tenth) cranial nerve supplies the heart. These fibers are distributed to the cardiac pacemakers, conducting tissue and to the myocardium. Vagal innervation to the SA node and AV junctional region is particularly important; vagal stimulation activates cholinergic receptors in the heart which exert strong inhibitory effects by slowing

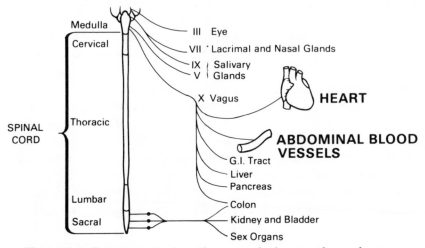

Figure 9-6. Parasympathetic pathways to the heart and vasculature.

heart rate and conduction velocity (Chapter 5) and by decreasing cardiac contractility, primarily of the atria (Chapter 6). As described later in this chapter, parasympathetic vasodilator fibers have been reported in vascular beds of the brain, myocardium, intestine, salivary glands and sex organs.

Preganglionic fibers of this division run to—or almost to—the innervated organs before synapsing so that parasympathetic effects tend to be more discrete and specific than sympathetic effects. Aside from its cardiovascular action, parasympathetic stimulation also induces contraction of non-vascular smooth muscle of bronchioles, gut and bladder, contraction of the pupil of the eye (miosis) and increased secretion of certain exocrine glands.

D. Vasoconstriction

Sympathetic vasoconstrictor impulses arise in the vasomotor center of the medulla as a result of either (a) intrinsic or extrinsic reflexes from various parts of the body, or (b) as descending impulses from the higher centers of the brain. The origin and nature of these two pathways will be discussed in Chapter 10. But however activated, sympathetic impulses will—as described above—promptly and almost simultaneously cause general constriction of the small arteries and veins.

However, all regions are not equally sensitive to constrictor impulses. Skin and muscle arteries show greater constriction at equivalent stimulation frequencies than do renal arteries (Fig. 9-7). The sensitivity of the vascular muscle is also influenced by metabolites so that during physical exercise, sympathetic stimulation will produce a lesser degree of constriction in skeletal muscle than it will at rest.

In addition to the action of arterial vasoconstriction (or dilation) on peripheral flow, there is an important effect on transcapillary pressure gradient and therefore on plasma volume. Hydrostatic pressure distal to the point of arterial constriction will be reduced; as a consequence there will be less filtration from and more reabsorption of tissue fluid into the capillaries (Chapter 8). In circulatory shock, for example, the increased vasoconstriction will notably increase the circulating plasma volume.

Fluid replacement is, however, a somewhat slower process than the vasomotor action itself; although vasoconstriction is well advanced

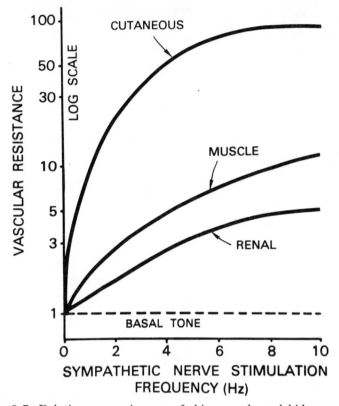

Figure 9-7. Relative responsiveness of skin, muscle and kidney vessels to vasoconstriction. Skin vessels show a greater increase in vascular resistance at equivalent stimulation frequencies. (From T. C. Ruch and H. D. Patton, *Physiology and Biophysics*. Philadelphia: W. B. Saunders Co., 1974.)

within 2 to 3 minutes after the onset of hypotension, the influx of fluid into the capillaries only begins after several minutes but continues for some hours afterward.

An important part of the sympathetic vascular response is *venocon-striction* which can significantly decrease venous capacitance and shift blood toward the heart, thus aiding venous return. At comparable levels of sympathetic stimulation frequency, venous vessels generally show a lesser degree of constriction than do the arterial vessels as indicated in Figure 9-8. This somewhat lesser responsiveness of the venous bed is probably advantageous, since it would prevent excessive rise in postcapillary resistance; a strong rise in capillary hydrostatic

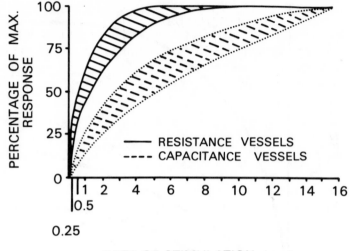

Figure 9-8. Frequency-response relationship of the resistance and capacitance vessels in the hindquarters of the cat. (From S. Mellander, *Acta Physiol. Scand.* 50:Suppl. 176, p. 1, 1960.)

pressure would lessen fluid reabsorption at the venous end of the capillary and tend to lower blood volume. Such a response would not be consistent with the general objective of sympathetic vasoconstriction which is to increase blood volume as well as arterial blood pressure.

Vascular beds differ in their relative contribution to the resistance/capacitance balance. As mentioned previously, skeletal muscle because of its bulk, is a large contributor to peripheral resistance; on the other hand, constriction of the splanchnic bed results in a substantial reduction of splanchnic venous capacitance and thus can be a significant factor in assisting venous return.

In summary, it should be noted that generalized vasoconstriction will usually have three vascular effects: (a) arteriolar constriction, which will increase vascular resistance, heighten the central arterial pressure and decrease flow to the constricted beds; (b) venoconstriction, which will reduce the caliber of the capacitance vessels and assist venous return; and (c) a reduction of capillary hydrostatic pressure with a resultant net increase in plasma volume.

E. Vasodilation

While vasoconstriction results only from sympathetic stimulation to alpha receptors, vasodilation is more complex and may be induced in several different ways, *e.g.*, by:

1. Inhibition of the Vasoconstrictor Center of the Medulla. This type of vasodilation may be the most common pathway and some investigators have questioned the existence of a true medullary vasodilator center.

2. Sympathetic Cholinergic (Muscarinic) Vasodilators. As previously mentioned, small arterial vessels in skeletal muscle are unique because they are innervated by sympathetic cholinergic vasodilator fibers which can be blocked by atropine. These receptors are activated only in unusual circumstances such as the "defense reaction" (Chapter 10).

3. Beta-sympathetic Vasodilators. These receptors are present primarily in skeletal muscle; when unmasked by alpha blockade, they respond with a mild, relatively transitory, vasodilation.

4. Parasympathetic Vasodilators. The activation of glossopharyngeal fibers to submaxillary salivary glands can evoke glandular secretions which ultimately result in the release of a neurohormone, bradykinin, which has a strong local vasodilator effect. In addition, sacral vasodilators to genital erectile tissue are important in reproduction; however, the remaining parasympathetic vasodilators play relatively minor roles.

F. Vascular Tone and the Abolition of Tone

Basal tone is the low level, continuous, active tension which exists in the vascular smooth muscle when it is at rest or under "basal" conditions. Even when deprived of all extrinsic neural or humoral influences, a measure of basal tone remains, due to the inherent action of the smooth muscle cells themselves, *i.e.*, the myogenic component of tone.

If the sympathetic constrictor fibers are intact, a somewhat higher level of continuous contractile activity is present due to low-frequency efferent impulses from the vasoconstrictor center of the medulla. Vasoconstrictor tone is not equal in the different tissues; it is highest in skeletal muscle, skin and in splanchnic vessels and least in vessels of the brain, myocardium and kidney. The degree of basal tone of neurogenic origin can be determined in experimental animals by severing of the vasoconstrictor fibers and measuring the change in blood flow and peripheral resistance.

Vascular tone is important in the continuous maintenance of arterial pressure. In case of severance of the spinal cord there will be a flaccid paralysis of all somatic motor elements below the transection (paraplegia); in addition, the sympathetic preganglionic vasoconstrictors will be interrupted and vasoconstrictor vascular tone to the entire body mass below the lesion will be lost. This usually results in a drastic fall in arterial pressure to levels of 60 to 80 mm Hg (spinal shock) partly because of the abrupt reduction of peripheral resistance and partly because of the loss of venoconstriction and decreased venous return.

A similar, though temporary and less severe fall in blood pressure results upon administration of an alpha adrenergic blocking agent such as phenoxybenzamine.

The higher the cord lesion, the more serious is the vascular disability. If the section is above the sixth thoracic segment, a condition of orthostatic hypotension usually exists; this means that if the patient is tilted to any type of head-up position, he will be unable to compensate for the gravity effect on the circulation by invoking the usual baroceptor reflexes (Chapter 13). The relatively inadequate orthostatic response of a patient with a cervical cord lesion compared to a patient with a lower thoracic cord lesion is illustrated in Figure 9-9.

Several days after spinal transection, vascular constriction begins a slow recovery, perhaps because of heightening of myogenic tone or the gradual establishment of spinal vascular reflexes. There also begins within a few days a denervation sensitivity of the vascular muscles involved. The vessels become abnormally sensitive to circulating or injected catecholamines so that local ischemia may develop. This phenomenon is usually more severe if the postganglionic (rather than preganglionic) fibers are interrupted. This effect is apparently due to the degeneration of the primary inactivating mechanism for catecholamines so that these substances reach unusually high concentrations at the local vascular nerve endings with resultant strong vascular constriction.

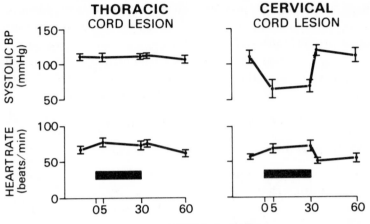

Figure 9-9. Effect of paraplegia on vascular responses to a posture change. *Black bars* indicate change from supine to sitting position. Patient with cervical cord lesion shows orthostatic fall in arterial pressure compared to patient with lower thoracic section. (From R. H. Johnson and J. M. K. Spalding, *Disorders of the Autonomic Nervous System.* Philadelphia: F. A. Davis Co., 1974.)

Humoral Control of Flow

Probably the most important humoral agents influencing flow are the *circulating catecholamines*; these may be (a) endogenous, *i.e.,* derived from the adrenal medulla or from excess catecholamines released at neural endings; or (b) exogenous, *e.g.,* administered by vein. In either case, the cardiovascular effects will be similar to those of sympathetic neural action. In severe exercise, circulatory shock or other forms of stress, the plasma concentration of catecholamines (epinephrine and norepinephrine) will increase markedly and reinforce the circulatory effects of sympathetic stimulation. However, the humoral catecholamines normally have only minor cardiovascular effects compared to those resulting from neural stimulation. Norepinephrine, the primary catecholamine, has a pure vasoconstrictor action in most beds. Epinephrine at low doses causes vasodilation through beta receptor stimulation but at high doses, its alpha constrictor effect overshadows the beta dilator action, particularly in skeletal muscle. The metabolic effects of sympathetic stimulation are due primarily to epinephrine.

Other humoral vasoactive substances circulating in the blood stream include angiotensin II, the most potent vasoconstrictor in the body, vasopressin, serotonin (5 hydroxytryptamine) and several prostaglandins. Except for the effect of prostaglandins on renal circulation (discussed in Chapter 15), the physiological role of these substances in normal cardiovascular regulation is not yet certain.

LOCAL REGULATION OF FLOW

Active Hyperemia

When tissues become metabolically more active e.g. exercise or if their temperature is raised, the microcirculatory vessels dilate and flow increases, a process known as active hyperemia. The mechanism of this effect is not certain but is thought to be a vasodilator action of accumulated metabolites such as CO_2 or lactic acid on the precapillary sphincters. The "metabolic" theory is strengthened by the fact that during severe exercise when skeletal muscle metabolism is at its peak and metabolic products such as CO_2 and lactic acid accumulate in the tissues, blood flow is very high.

Other metabolites such as K^+ and H^+ as well as decreased Po_2 and increased osmolality have also been proposed as primary dilator agents. There is increasing evidence that the responsible metabolite may vary with the tissue involved; in the hypoxic myocardium, *e.g.*, adenosine and some of its related compounds have been implicated as the active agents. In the salivary gland, bradykinin, and in the kidney, renin and prostaglandins are known to have strong local vascular effects. However, some of the evidence is conflicting and further investigation is needed in this important field.

Reactive Hyperemia

If blood flow to a part is arrested by arterial occlusion for a period of a few seconds to several minutes, the flow upon release will exceed the control flow for a short period before returning to preocclusion levels. This excess afterflow is known as "reactive hyperemia" and as indicated in Figure 9-10, the resulting degree and duration of the overshoot are roughly proportional to the duration of the occlusion.

Tissues differ in their reactive hyperemic response; heart and brain show large responses, skeletal muscle intermediate and liver, lung and

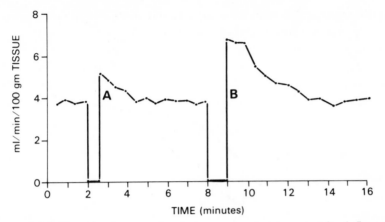

Figure 9-10. Reactive hyperemia. *A,* temporary increase in blood flow to forearm after 30-second occlusion. After 60-second occlusion, *B,* the reactive flow is of greater magnitude and duration.

skin the least. The cause of the increased flow is not clear but the relation between the length of occlusion and degree of hyperemia suggests that either oxygen lack in the tissues or the accumulation of metabolites is responsible. Reactive hyperemia will result after ischemia (partial or full occlusion of arterial supply) or hypoxia (reduced Po_2 in the tissue).

Autoregulation

If individual organs are perfused with blood at different pressures so that flow-pressure relations can be studied, the initial response in almost all cases resembles *curve A,* Figure 9-11. In some tissues, particularly kidney, brain and heart, the flow will change within 30 to 60 seconds to an "autoregulatory" adaptation such as *curve B* (Fig. 9-11), in which there is a tendency to maintain the local blood flow relatively constant in the face of fluctuating pressures. Some tissues such as skin and lung show minimal autoregulation.

Curve A is a passive type of curve and its exponential nature is due mainly to the constantly increasing diameter which occurs in a flexible tube when subjected to increasing transmural pressure (Chapter 2). During autoregulation (*curve B*), the higher flows are achieved at low pressure by relaxation of the vascular muscle, and the lower flows at higher pressures by constriction. The net result—the maintenance of

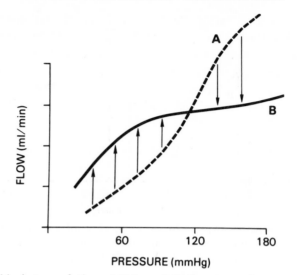

Figure 9-11. Autoregulation of kidney. Initial pressure-flow response curve (A) changes to a plateau-type curve (B) within 30 to 60 seconds.

a relatively stable flow—is particularly advantageous to vital organs such as brain and heart; in case of hypotension or failing circulation, local flow will increase. In case of higher pressure, excess flow will be reduced.

Those organs with the smallest neurogenic tone, *i.e.*, brain, heart and kidney, show the highest autoregulatory ability; conversely tissues with the highest resting vascular tone, *e.g.*, skin, have the least auto-regulatory ability. Although the ability to autoregulate is affected to some extent by neural and humoral influences such as vasoconstrictor tone and pH of the blood, the autoregulatory response is largely intrinsic and occurs when tissues are fully denervated and isolated; it is, therefore, essentially a local phenomenon.

Different explanations have been advanced for autoregulation; one of these, the myogenic theory, suggests that increased perfusion pressure increases the muscle tension in the vessel wall, stimulating it to contract and thus reduce flow; with reduction in perfusion pressure, there is relaxation of the wall and increase in vessel caliber. This theory proposes, therefore, that distension of the muscle is the self-regulating mediator.

Other investigators believe that autoregulation is associated with the state of oxygenation of the tissue; a decrease in flow will produce a decrease in local tissue P_{O_2} and an increase in tissue P_{CO_2}; the decreased P_{O_2} theoretically relaxes the precapillary sphincter and the flow would again rise. With restored flow, the P_{O_2} and P_{CO_2} levels are returned toward normal as shown in Figure 9-12. Regardless of the validity of any specific theory, it seems very likely that the balance of tissue flow is maintained in some manner similar to the negative feedback mechanism shown in Figure 9-12.

LONG-TERM REGULATION OF BLOOD FLOW

The previous portions of this chapter relate to rapid adjustments of the circulation. But what are the responses if demands for additional flow are built up more gradually? If, for example, the main arterial supply to a part of the body such as skin or muscle is gradually occluded, the pressure and flow in the distal vessel will be reduced. What is the response of the tissue to such a situation? In tissues with adequate collateral circulation, e.g., skeletal muscle, collateral vessels will dilate over the ensuing days and weeks so that total arterial flow to the part will gradually be restored to near normal. Thus the local circulatory demand has in some way instigated an increased blood supply. This type of adaptation is, however, severely restricted in tissues such as brain or kidney in which collateral vessels are minimal or absent; in such cases an infarct (area of necrosis) is likely with degeneration, loss of function and replacement fibrosis occurring in at least a portion of the involved area. The question of myocardial infarct is discussed in Chapter 14.

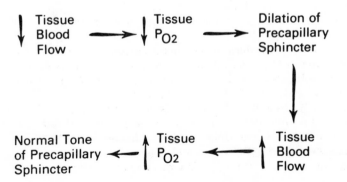

Figure 9-12. Possible mechanism for autoregulation of tissue blood flow involving effect of altered P_{O_2} on precapillary sphincter tone.

On the other hand, if arterial pressure and flow to a part is excessive, *e.g.*, in arteries above the level at which partial occlusion of the abdominal aorta has been produced in an experimental animal, the flow to tissues above the occlusion level will at first be excessive because of the hypertension in this portion of the arterial tree. Gradually, however, the flow to the involved regions will return to normal by virtue of gradually increased constriction of the arteries and arterioles in the area. Thus, if blood flow is artificially increased or decreased, it will, if left alone, tend to gradually return to previous control levels. Similar circulatory responses occur with alterations of oxygen supply. Prolonged hypoxia will stimulate increased flow and in embryonic or fetal tissue will promote the generation of new blood vessels.

It appears, therefore, that the relation of flow to tissue metabolism is the dominant factor in the long-term regulation of blood flow. It seems likely that the mechanism of this effect is either *via* oxygen demand or through an oxygen-linked metabolite. But how oxygen lack actually brings about increased flow or vascular architectural expansion is not known. The increased physical stretch and tension of vasodilation on growth potential of vascular cells may be a factor; regardless of the actual cause, however, it is known that the vascular cells of younger tissue are more responsive to growth stimuli of hypoxia and ischemia than are those of older tissue.

REFERENCES

BARCROFT, H.: Circulation in skeletal muscle. In *Handbook of Physiology*, Section 2: *Circulation*, vol. II, ed. by W. F. Hamilton and P. Dow. Washington, D. C.: American Physiological Society, 1963.

JOHANSSON, B.: Vascular reactivity in hypertension. Symposium. *Fed. Proc.* 33:121–149, 1974.

JOHNSON, P. C.: Principles of peripheral circulatory control. In *Peripheral Circulation*, ed. by P. C. Johnson. New York: John Wiley & Sons, 1978.

JOHNSON, R. H., AND J. M. K. SPALDING: *Disorders of the Autonomic Nervous System*. Philadelphia: F. A. Davis Co., 1974.

KOELLE, G. B.: Neurohumoral transmission and the autonomic nervous system. In *Pharmacological Basis of Therapeutics*, 5th ed., ed. by L. S. Goodman and A. Gilman. New York: Macmillan Co., 1975.

MELLANDER, S., AND B. JOHANSSON: Control of resistance, exchange and capacitance functions in the peripheral circulation. *Pharmacol. Rev.* 20:117–196, 1968.

RANDALL, W. C. (Ed.): *Neural Regulation of the Heart.* New York: Oxford University Press, 1977.

SHEPHERD, J. T.: *Physiology of the Circulation in Human Limbs in Health and Disease.* Philadelphia: W. B. Saunders Co., 1963.

SLEIGHT, P.: Drugs acting on the heart. In *Circulation of the Blood,* ed. by D. G. James. Baltimore: University Park Press, 1978.

STAINSBY, W. N.: Local control of regional blood flow. *Annu. Rev. Physiol.* 35: 151, 1973.

chapter 10

Regulation of Arterial Blood Pressure

ARTERIAL PRESSURE REGULATION—GENERAL PRINCIPLES

The method by which arterial pressure is regulated depends upon whether short-term or long-term adaptation is required. Short-term adjustments (over minutes and hours) are intended to correct temporary imbalances of pressure such as those caused by postural change, exercise or hemorrhage. Whatever the inciting cause, the reaction is usually a series of rapid autonomic reflex responses mediated *via* the cardiovascular centers of the medulla.

Long-term arterial pressure adjustments (weeks or months) are usually concerned with the balance between extracellular fluid and blood volume on the one hand and renal mechanisms controlling urinary output on the other. The latter particularly involves pituitary-adrenal cortical mechanisms which control water and sodium excretion by the kidney; disturbances of this process may result in gradual increase in arterial pressure and, if continued, in enduring hypertension.

Arterial blood pressure, because it determines blood flow, is probably the most important controlled variable in the circulatory system. We know from the general hemodynamic equation discussed in Chapter 2 that blood pressure is, in effect, the mathematical product of cardiac output and peripheral resistance; the cardiovascular centers control the arterial pressure through adjustments of these two variables. However, these centers are themselves governed by reflex responses to pressure changes and by impulses from higher neural centers. Thus the arterial pressure, acting through classical feedback mechanisms, is both the controlled and controlling variable (Fig. 10-1).

This chapter is concerned primarily with how the cardiovascular

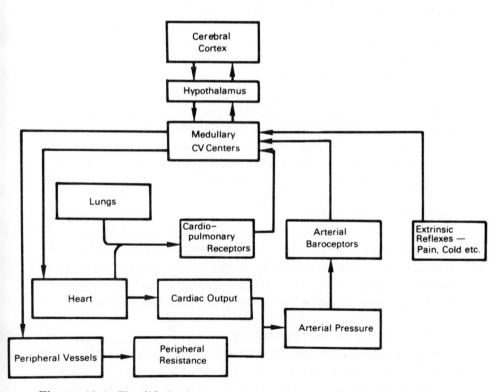

Figure 10-1. Simplified schema showing primary pathways for short-term regulation of arterial blood pressure.

centers interact with the cardiac output and peripheral resistance in the process of regulating the arterial pressure.

CARDIOVASCULAR CENTERS OF THE MEDULLA

The main nervous control of the circulation resides in several functionally diverse areas or "centers" in the dorsal reticular matter of the medulla, which are collectively known as cardiovascular (CV) centers; together with the respiratory center, with which they have close neural connection, these are the "vital nervous centers" whose integrity is absolutely essential for survival of the organism. There are two major divisions of the cardiovascular control area, *i.e.*, the cardiac and vasomotor, which are concerned with the neural control of the heart and peripheral blood vessels respectively. These two areas are not well defined so that there is both anatomical and functional overlap between them. Careful animal experiments involving surgical transection as well as microelectrode stimulation and functional mapping have indicated that both the cardiac and vasomotor areas have, in turn, further subdivisions with specialized functions.

One of the clearest entities in the cardiac area is a "cardioinhibitory center" located in the nucleus ambiguus and dorsal nucleus of the vagus nerve. Vagal efferents from these sites carry impulses which act primarily to decrease heart rate and to a lesser degree the contractility of the atria. The existence of a corollary sympathetic "cardiostimulatory center" in the lateral medulla has been reported but is less certain; cardiac stimulation is probably achieved mainly through lesser activity of the cardioinhibitory center than through heightened activity of a cardiostimulatory center.

The "vasomotor center" of the medulla consists, in most species, of a lateral "vasoconstrictor area" whose neurons descend in the spinal cord and synapse with cells of the intermediolateral cell column. Their preganglionic fibers are responsible for the widespread sympathetic vasoconstriction described in Chapter 9. The "vasodilator area" is more questionable and it is probable that vasodilation is mainly due to inhibition of the vasoconstrictor center.

The close proximity of these centers to each other and their tendency to function in a coordinated fashion in the interests of arterial pressure control have led to the characterization of the lateral and superior portions of the CV center area as the "pressor area," and the more medial as the "depressor area" (Fig. 10-2). In most species, stimulation of the pressor area will induce both an increase in cardiac rate and contractility and a generalized increase in peripheral resistance while depressor area stimulation usually elicits the reverse. The "vasoconstrictor," "cardiostimulatory," and "cardioinhibitory" areas are tonically active, *i.e.*, they emit, even at rest, a constant low level of efferent impulses so that cutting of these efferent fibers will eliminate vasoconstrictor, cardiac stimulatory and cardioinhibitory effects respectively on the target organs.

The various CV centers usually function reciprocally, *i.e.*, when vagal slowing is initiated by the cardioinhibitory center, there is simultaneously reduced activity of the cardiostimulatory center. While the medullary cardiovascular centers are key factors in regulating the circulation, they are not fully autonomous. The CV centers are, for example, subject to descending impulses from higher centers such as the hypothalamus and cerebral cortex; furthermore, the target organs themselves have some degree of autonomy. As previously discussed, the myocardium is capable of intrinsic heterometric adjustments (Chapter 6) and individual organs are capable of autoregulation which is independent of nervous control (Chapter 9).

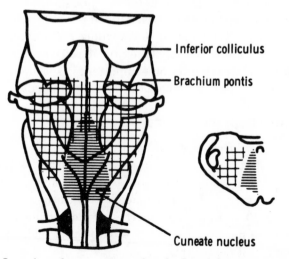

Figure 10-2. Location of pressor (*crosshatched*) and depressor (*horizontally lined*) areas in the brain stem of the cat. (From J. Alexander, *Neurophysiology* 9:205, 1946.)

INTRINSIC REFLEXES OF THE CARDIOVASCULAR SYSTEM

"Intrinsic" reflexes, that is those which originate from within the circulatory system itself, are usually distinguished from "extrinsic" or those originating in other systems or organs. The intrinsic reflexes, by far the more important in the short-term regulation of blood pressure, are for the most part activated by special receptors; these receptors are usually sensitive to pressure or to special chemical stimuli. Those sensitive to pressure are termed stretch receptors, pressoceptors or mechanoceptors, but more commonly "baroceptors." The "chemoreceptors" of the vascular system are primarily concerned with respiratory regulation but may in certain circumstances play a secondary role in circulatory control.

A large number of cardiovascular reflexes have been described and through animal experimentation their pathways have been at least partly traced; however, their actual functional role in the intact human circulation is often difficult to determine. Our present knowledge, while admittedly incomplete, does, however, permit a few generalizations regarding reflex control of the circulation. These are that (a) the high-pressure, arterial baroceptors of the carotid sinus and aortic arch are by far the key reflexes in short-term regulation of the circulation, (b) the cardiopulmonary baroceptors (all low pressure except those of the left ventricle) while not yet as well defined as the arterial baroceptors, seem to act mainly to temper and modulate the carotid and aortic baroceptor responses, and (c) the extrinsic reflexes play a minor role in ordinary regulation but become important in specific situations, *e.g.*, in severe somatic pain or sudden distension of the gut.

Arterial Baroceptors

Afferent fibers from specialized pressure-sensitive endings in the walls of the aortic arch and internal carotid arteries travel *via* the aortic and carotid sinus nerves, join the vagus and glossopharyngeal nerves respectively, and make connections with the CV centers of the medulla (Fig. 10-3). Impulses from the carotid and aortic chemoreceptors, which are near their respective baroceptor endings, travel over the same afferent nerves (Fig. 10-3).

Stretching of the baroceptor endings generates action potentials in the afferent nerves (Fig. 10-4) whose frequency is approximately proportional to the pressure change in the artery.

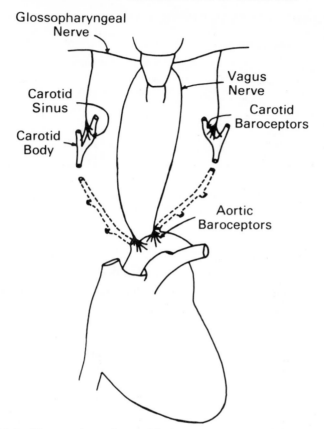

Glossopharyngeal
Nerve

Vagus
Nerve

Carotid
Sinus

Carotid
Baroceptors

Carotid
Body

Aortic
Baroceptors

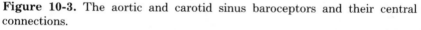

Figure 10-3. The aortic and carotid sinus baroceptors and their central connections.

The high pressure baroceptors respond to absolute stretch, *i.e.*, to changes in the arterial transmural pressure but even more strongly to the rate of change of pressure, *i.e.*, dP/dt. The baroceptor response is greatest in the physiological range of blood pressure (80 to 150 mm Hg) and there is some evidence that the carotid receptors are somewhat more sensitive than the aortic (Fig. 10-5).

The baroceptors are particularly important in maintaining adequate pressure (and, therefore, flow) to the brain and heart during ordinary circulatory stresses such as postural changes and elevated intrathoracic pressure which tend to decrease venous return and arterial pressure.

It should be noted that in common with most reflexes which stabilize a controlled variable, the aortic baroceptor reflex involves negative

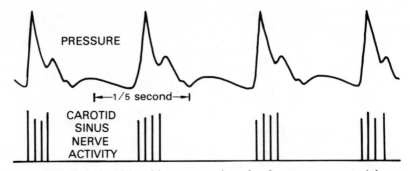

Figure 10-4. Relationship of baroceptor impulse frequency to arterial pressure. Carotid arterial blood pressure shown above and impulses in the carotid sinus nerve below. (From D. W. Bronk and G. Stella, *Am. J. Physiol.* 110:708, 1935.)

feedback. This means that *increased* arterial pressure at the baroceptor site will increase the frequency of afferent impulses in the aortic and carotid sinus nerves. This stimulus results in greater activity in the medullary depressor area and inhibition of the pressor area so that

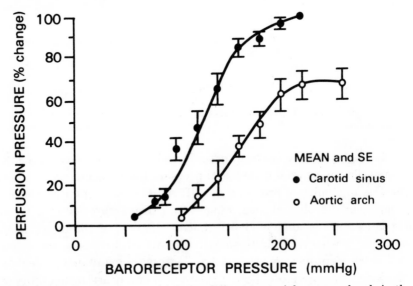

Figure 10-5. Baroceptor sensitivity at different arterial pressure levels in the dog. At equivalent pressures the carotid baroceptors were more sensitive than the aortic receptors. (From D. E. Donald and A. J. Edis, *J. Physiol.* 215:521, 1971.)

heart rate and myocardial contractility are *decreased* and vasoconstrictor and venoconstrictor tone are *lessened* (Fig. 10-6). Thus the increased blood pressure leads to reflex action aimed at reducing the pressure back toward normal level (depressor reflex); if baroceptor stretch is decreased, the afferent impulse frequency is decreased and the reverse response occurs (pressor reflex).

As suggested by Figure 10-5, at higher arterial pressure levels, the baroceptors transmit fewer impulses, which may be due to lesser deformation of the endings at the higher pressures. In chronic hypertension, the baroceptors continue to function but are "reset" at a higher level which then becomes the baseline for further baroceptor response. There is some evidence to indicate that arterial baroceptors normally respond more actively to a decrease in pressure than to an increase, *i.e.*, are more effective in combatting acute hypotension than acute hypertension.

In general the strength of the baroceptor reflex decrees that in most short-term situations, there is a reciprocal relationship between arterial blood pressure and heart rate. However, this does not universally hold. For example, during static (isometric) exercise, systolic and diastolic blood pressures and heart rate all increase progressively (Chapter 12). In the diving (face immersion) reflex, there is a sharp decrease in both arterial pressure and heart rate (Chapter 13) and during the "defense reaction" (described later in this chapter) there is a pronounced increase in arterial pressure as well as in heart rate. It may be that supramedullary centers, which are involved in all three of these instances, may be responsible for the temporary inhibition of the baroreflexes.

Decreased responsiveness of the arterial baroreflexes has been reported as occurring with advancing age, in hypertension and in coro-

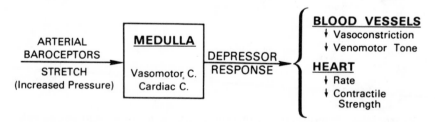

Figure 10-6. Hemodynamic response to arterial baroceptor stimulation.

nary heart disease. It has been suggested that arteriosclerotic changes in the arterial walls with decreased compliance may make the receptors less sensitive to deformation; however, further investigation is needed in this area.

Cardiopulmonary (CP) Reflexes

Cardiopulmonary receptors are intrathoracic sensors, most of which are located at low pressure sites in the walls of the heart, great vessels and lungs. CP reflexes are complex but because of their broad functional role have been the focus of increasing research interest. They are usually classified on the basis of location, *i.e.*, (a) atrial and vena caval, (b) ventricular, and (c) pulmonary (Fig. 10-7).

A. Atrial and Vena Caval Receptors. These are low-pressure receptors whose impulses travel mainly *via* large, medullated (fast-conducting) vagal fibers. When distended by increased venous return, the usual cardiac result is a heightened sympathetic activity with an accompanying tachycardia (*Bainbridge reflex*). The circulatory response is a minor one, however, compared to the renal effect; the efferent sympathetic traffic to the kidney is decreased with a resulting increase in urine flow. Current evidence suggests that increased left atrial stretch inhibits the release of the antidiuretic hormone (ADH)

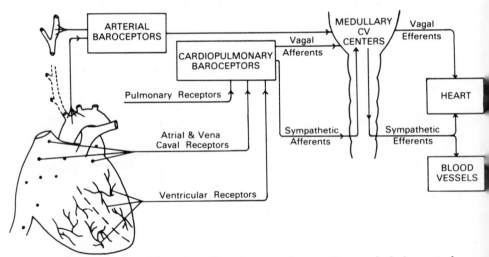

Figure 10-7. Arterial and cardiopulmonary baroceptors and their central connections.

from the posterior pituitary gland, and that right atrial stretch reduces renin secretion from the kidney; both of these reflex effects, induced by increased "fullness" of the circulatory system, tend to increase urinary output and reduce plasma volume. Although these endings respond to stretch, they are, because of their functional role, sometimes called "volume receptors."

B. *Ventricular Receptors.* These sensors, because of their location in the walls of the left ventricle are the only high-pressure receptors in the group. When stimulated by increased stretch, afferent impulses from ventricular receptors travel *via* small, non-medullated (slow-conducting) vagal fibers to the medulla and elicit a bradycardia and vasodilation, *i.e.*, a depressor response.

A peculiar characteristic of these receptors is that a very similar, hypotensive response is produced by injection into the heart or coronary circulation of a specific chemical agent, called veratrine (an alkaloid extract from lilacs). This unusual chemoceptor response, known as the *Bezold-Jarisch reflex*, may also be triggered by intra-coronary injections of a contrast medium during coronary angiography and by the accumulation of metabolites under certain pathological conditions. The hypotensive reaction in cardiogenic shock produced by coronary occlusion may be partly due to activation of these ventricular receptors.

The above-described responses from stimulation of ventricular receptors are the result of afferent impulses which travel *via* the vagus nerves. Ventricular distension in experimental animals will also stimulate sympathetic afferent endings in the ventricle which will invoke strong arterial pressor responses as well as alterations in respiration. The physiological and pathological significance of these sympathetic ventricular CP reflexes is not clear at present.

C. *Pulmonary Receptors.* A variety of reflexes arising from the lung are known to be important in the control of respiration but their circulatory significance in man is still uncertain. However, pulmonary congestion which occurs during severe exercise or increased pulmonary venous pressure may activate juxtapulmonary receptors (so called J receptors) and induce reflex tachycardia and dyspnea (difficulty in breathing).

D. *Cardiopulmonary Inhibitory Reflex.* An important observation reported by Shepherd and Donald and their colleagues is the inhibitory effect of some CP vagal afferent nerves (receptor site as yet unknown) on sympathetic vasoconstriction and heart rate. When these vagal fibers are interrupted, there is an increase in heart rate and general vasoconstriction as well as an increase in renin release. Corollary studies have shown that an increase in central blood volume, *e.g.*, by large intravenous fluid infusions will cause a decrease in the systemic vascular resistance. The CP inhibitory reflex is most marked at lower levels of arterial pressure when the aortic baroceptors are less active. Thus it appears that this CP inhibitory reflex (activated by the low-pressure CP receptors) has a function generally similar to that of the arterial baroceptor reflex and acts in concert with it.

Arterial Chemoreceptors

These special endings, located in the carotid and aortic bodies (near the carotid sinus and aortic arch receptors) respond to a reduction in arterial Po_2, an increase in Pco_2 or an increase in arterial H^+ concentration, with hyperventilation, sympathetic vasoconstriction (mainly in skeletal muscle) and bradycardia (vagal). While the main purpose of the arterial chemoreceptor reflex is to stimulate respiratory minute volume, its secondary circulatory effects appear to be aimed at increasing oxygen delivery to the brain and heart through general peripheral vasoconstriction and increased arterial pressure. The chemoreceptor reflex becomes a protective factor in certain pathophysiological situations such as the hypoxia of altitude (low arterial Po_2) and circulatory shock (peripheral ischemia).

EXTRINSIC REFLEXES

Certain stimuli originating outside the circulation may invoke cardiovascular responses *via* somatic afferent pathways. The central connections are not known and the responses are usually less consistent than in the case of the intrinsic reflexes described above. Among the more common of these extrinsic reflexes are:

Pain

Pain produces a somewhat variable hemodynamic response. Mild to moderate pain usually elicits increased arterial pressure and tachycardia. Severe pain, as might be experienced by undue stretching of the gall bladder, intestine or ureter, or deep trauma to a bone or joint, may induce bradycardia, hypotension and sometimes circulatory collapse and fainting. Overly-rapid evacuation of a markedly distended hollow organ may also cause reflex hypotension and sometimes circulatory collapse. This reflex is responsible for the clinical admonition that if pressure in over-distended organs such as the stomach or urinary bladder is relieved by intubation or catheterization, the decompression should be done slowly.

Cold

Somatic afferent fibers from cutaneous thermosensitive endings travel to the hypothalamus and reflexly induce cutaneous vasoconstriction and piloerection (erection of hair). Intense local cold, *e.g.*, by immersion of one hand to the wrist in ice water for 1 minute (the "*cold pressor*" *test*) will result in an increase in arterial pressure through stimulation of pain as well as cold receptors.

It has been reported that in some patients with coronary heart disease, the cold pressor test increases coronary artery resistance, decreases coronary blood flow and sometimes precipitates angina (chest pain); these changes did not occur in normal subjects (Fig. 10-8). The cause of the angina is not certain but may be due either to

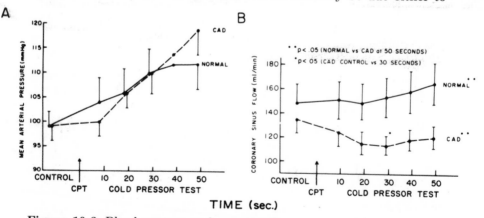

Figure 10-8. Blood pressure and coronary flow responses of patients with coronary artery disease (CAD) and normal subjects to the cold pressor test. *A* indicates similar arterial pressure response in the two groups, and *B*, a decrease in coronary flow in the patients. *Arrow* indicates start of 50-second cold pressor test. (Reprinted by permission from G. H. Mudge, W. Grossman, R. M. Mills, M. Lesch, and E. Braunwald, *N. Engl. J. Med.* 295:1333, 1976.)

reflex coronary vasoconstriction or a relative myocardial ischemia due
to the increased aortic afterload.

Special Somatic Reflexes

Strong somatic afferent stimulation may cause circulatory responses,
particularly of the depressor type. *Rapid angular acceleration* (rota-
tion or spinning of the body on its own axis) will, for example, induce
excessive afferent stimulation from the labyrinth of the inner ear and
may cause nausea, vomiting and a depressor reflex. The *oculocardiac
reflex* refers to bradycardia and hypotension induced by lateral pressure on the eyeball; the latter reflex, by virtue of its efferent vagal
path, is sometimes effective in aborting attacks of cardiac arrhythmias
such as atrial fibrillation (Chapter 5).

HIGHER CENTER INFLUENCES

CNS Ischemic Response

Apart from the baroceptor response induced by a fall in blood
pressure, severe hypotension, such as occurs in circulatory shock, will
result in a profound, generalized vasoconstriction. Since the mechanism of this powerful reflex is probably hypoxia or ischemia of the
brain stem, it is known as the "CNS ischemic response." It apparently
represents a "last ditch" effort to maintain adequate perfusion of the
CV medullary centers and is activated only when the arterial pressure
is reduced to levels of about 50 to 70 mm Hg.

A similar mechanism is thought to be operative in the "Cushing
reflex," which is a marked hypertension following acute elevation of
cerebrospinal fluid (CSF) pressure; in this instance the flow of blood
to the brain stem is decreased by the external pressure of CSF fluid on
the blood vessels, thus activating the CNS ischemic response. The
arterial blood pressure rises progressively in the effort to exceed the
CSF pressure and maintain adequate blood flow to the brain.

Role of the Hypothalamus

The hypothalamus, as a midway point between the cerebral cortex
and the medulla, provides a level of integration for a number of
essential cardiovascular activities. Among these are the coordination
of responses to emotion, exercise and temperature change. Experimen-

tal animals with lesions in the ventromedial hypothalamus will, upon relatively slight provocation, react with intense rage associated with high blood pressure, sweating and pupillary dilation. The hypothalamus plays a key role in determining the circulatory and other autonomic responses which accompany swings of mood and emotion.

The efficient and effective performance of *physical exercise* or work requires a close integration of the circulation and metabolism. That this is done by the hypothalamus is suggested by the fact that stimulation of the fields of Forel will, in the dog, produce a series of autonomic reactions closely resembling those which accompany physical exercise; these include highly coordinated responses of dilation of skeletal muscle vessels, constriction of non-muscle beds and release of plasma catecholamines into the blood (Chapter 12, Physical Exercise).

The control center for *temperature regulation*, located in the preoptic region of the anterior hypothalamus, plays a key role in balancing heat production and loss. When the body (or the hypothalamus) is heated, sympathetic vasoconstrictor impulse traffic is decreased, vascular smooth muscles are relaxed, the cutaneous arteriovenous anastomoses (AVAs) of exposed areas are opened and sweating occurs; all of these are essential to the preservation of heat balance. With cold the reverse response occurs in order to reduce heat loss (Chapter 11, Cutaneous Circulation).

Corticohypothalamic Patterns—Defense Reaction

From a circulatory standpoint, one of the more important behavior patterns involving the cerebral cortex and the hypothalamus is the "defense reaction." It has been shown that stimulation of a localized area in the ventral hypothalamus of the cat will produce circulatory reactions very similar to those invoked by the presence of actual danger or threat of danger to the animal. These reactions include sympathetic cholinergic vasodilation of skeletal muscle (to permit immediate maximum muscular effort), generalized sympathetic vasoconstriction and elevation of arterial pressure, increased plasma catecholamines and increased rate and contractility of the heart. These changes, similar to those mentioned as preparation for muscular exercise, instantly prepare the animal for full scale "fight or flight" reaction.

It has also been observed that stimulation of another hypothalamic site, the depressor area, located very near the defense center, calls forth a strong sympathetic inhibition involving hypotension and brady-cardia; this sympathoinhibition resembles the "playing dead" reaction used by certain animals as a protective measure and is thought to be involved in psychogenic fainting. It has been suggested that in the face of overpowering stress, the corticohypothalamic depressor response may offer, in addition to fight or flight, a third option, *i.e.*, fainting and oblivion (Chapter 13, Fainting). The pathways involved in the defense reaction and the depressor reaction are shown in Figure 10-9.

LONG-TERM REGULATION OF ARTERIAL BLOOD PRESSURE

The previous portions of this chapter have been concerned with relatively short-term regulation of blood pressure. Guyton has recently advanced the concept that long-term control has a very different basis, namely the blood volume-urinary output balance, which in turn, is mainly influenced by the renin-angiotensin-aldosterone system (Fig. 10-10).

As indicated in Figure 10-10, an increase in arterial pressure, ①, causes increased fluid output through the kidneys, and a reduction in extracellular fluid volume, ③, blood volume, ④, and venous return, ⑥. The subsequent decrease in cardiac output will act to reduce the arterial pressure.

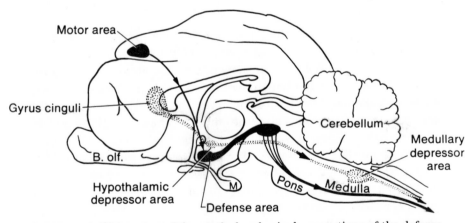

Figure 10-9. Illustration of the cortical and spinal connections of the defense center and "depressor area" of the hypothalamus. (From B. Folkow and E. Neil, *Circulation*. London: Oxford University Press, 1971.)

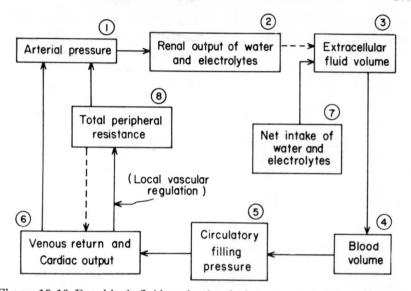

Figure 10-10. Renal-body fluid mechanism for long-term regulation of arterial blood pressure. (From A. C. Guyton, *Textbook of Medical Physiology,* 5th ed. Philadelphia: W. B. Saunders Co., 1976.)

The continuous and overriding nature of this mechanism is due to two important factors: (a) only very small changes in body fluid volume are required to produce marked changes in arterial pressure; and (b) the kidney-body fluid control system has infinite gain. The latter implies that if atherosclerosis or some other process heightened renal vascular resistance, the arterial pressure would rise to whatever degree required to generate the necessary urinary output.

In Chapter 9, evidence was presented that both short- and long-term blood flow regulation are dictated by metabolic needs of the tissue and in the case of cardiac output, of the body as a whole. Thus the heart does not control its own output but merely pumps—within its capability—whatever blood is brought to it.

Guyton's interesting concept has the further implication that cardiac output and arterial pressure are separate entities, controlled by different mechanisms and are, in a sense, independent variables. Thus, an elevated blood pressure may be initiated by the need for ample perfusion through a renal bed in order to maintain urinary output; on the other hand, the hypertension may endure because of the increased peripheral resistance needed for the tissues to autoregulate their flow at an acceptably low level. Guyton's theory offers at present one of the more plausible explanations for long-term circulatory regulation of blood pressure.

REFERENCES

ABBOUD, F. M., D. D. HEISTAD, A. L. MARK, AND P. G. SCHMID: Reflex control of the peripheral circulation. *Prog. Cardiovasc. Dis.* 18 (No. 5):371–403, 1976.

GUYTON, A. C., T. G. COLEMAN, AND H. J. GRANGER: Circulation: Overall regulation. *Annu. Rev. Physiol.* 34:13–46, 1972.

GUYTON, A. C., A. W. COWLEY, D. B. YOUNG, T. G. COLEMAN, J. E. HALL, AND J. W. DeCLUE: Integration and control of circulatory function. In *Cardiovascular Physiology II*, vol. 9, International Review of Physiology, ed. by A. C. Guyton and A. W. Cowley. Baltimore: University Park Press, 1976.

HILTON, S. M.: Hypothalamic regulation of the cardiovascular system. *Br. Med. Bull.* 22:243, 1966.

KIRCHHEIM, H. R.: Systemic arterial baroceptor reflexes. *Physiol. Rev.* 56:100, 1976.

KOSTREVA, D. R., G. L. HESS, E. J. ZUPERKU, J. NEUMARK, R. L. COON, AND J. P. KAMPINE: Cardiac responses to stimulation of thoracic afferents in the primate and canine. *Am. J. Physiol.* 231:1279–1284, 1976.

LÖFVING, B.: Cardiovascular adjustments induced from the rostral cingulate gyrus. *Acta Physiol. Scand.* 53:Suppl. 184, 1961.

MANCIA, G., R. R. LORENZ, AND J. T. SHEPHERD: Reflex control of circulation by heart and lungs. In *Cardiovascular Physiology II,* International Review of Physiology, ed. by A. C. Guyton and A. W. Cowley. Baltimore: University Park Press, 1976.

RANDALL, W. C.: *Neural Regulation of the Heart.* New York: Oxford University Press, 1977.

SAGAWA, K., M. KUMADA, AND L. P. SCHRAMM: Nervous control of the circulation. In *Cardiovascular Physiology,* MTP International Review of Sciences, ed. by A. C. Guyton and C. E. Jones. Baltimore: University Park Press, 1974.

SEAGARD, J. L., H. J. PEDERSON, D. R. KOSTREVA, D. L. VAN HORN, J. F. CUSICK, AND J. P. KAMPINE: Ultrastructural identification of afferent fibers in cardiac nerves. *Am. J. Anat.* 153:217–232, 1979.

chapter **11**

Circulation to Special Regions

CEREBRAL CIRCULATION

Anatomy

The main arteries to the cerebrum—the anterior, middle and posterior cerebral—come off the circle of Willis, which in turn is derived

181

from the basilar and internal carotid arteries. Branches of the vertebrals and proximal basilar artery supply the cerebellum and base of the brain (Fig. 11-1).

The blood vessels traverse the subarachnoid space before penetrating the brain substance. Venous drainage is *via* the superficial venous intradural sinuses of the cranium which empty primarily into the internal jugular vein; the wall support of the dural sinuses helps prevent their collapse when subjected to negative transmural pressure upon standing (Chapter 4).

Cerebrospinal Fluid (CSF)

The CSF, which has a total volume of about 150 ml, is formed in the choroid plexuses of the four ventricles at a rate of 400 to 600 ml/day; it circulates freely between the ventricles and cisterns of the brain, the subarachnoid space and the central canal of the spinal cord (Fig. 11-2). Originating as a plasma filtrate, it becomes CSF through facilitated

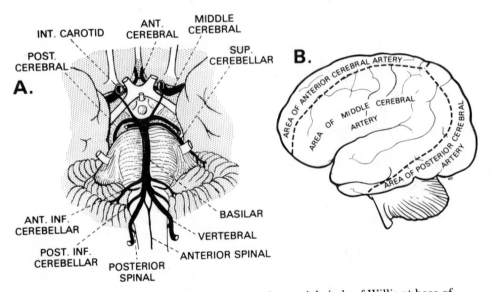

Figure 11-1. Arterial supply to the brain. *A,* arterial circle of Willis at base of the brain is formed by the basilar and internal carotid arteries. *B,* approximate area of distribution of the three main arteries to the cerebral hemispheres. (From E. Gardner, *Fundamentals of Neurology.* Philadelphia: W. B. Saunders Co., 1963.)

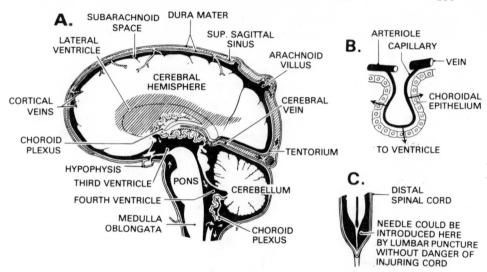

Figure 11-2. Circulation of cerebrospinal fluid (CSF). *A,* median section of the brain with projection of one lateral ventricle (oblique lines), the 3rd and 4th ventricles, central canal of the cord and subarachnoid space. CSF is formed from blood plasma and choroidal epithelium, *B,* passes into the ventricles and ultimately drains into the dural sinuses *via* the arachnoidal villi, *A.* (From E. Gardner, *Fundamentals of Neurology.* Philadelphia: W. B. Saunders Co., 1963.)

diffusion, active transport and secretion, the last being an energy-requiring process of the choroidal epithelium (Fig. 11-2*B*); it differs from blood serum mainly in its very small protein content (20 to 40 mg/100 ml) compared to that of serum (5500 to 8000 mg/100 ml). Protein content of CSF is, however, diagnostically useful since it is increased in multiple sclerosis, spinal canal blockade and brain tumors.

CSF is usually obtained *via* lumbar puncture (Fig. 11-2*C*). It has a normal pressure of 120 to 180 mm H$_2$O which represents a balance between its rate of formation and absorption back into the blood stream. Reabsorption is mainly *via* arachnoidal villi which invaginate the dural sinuses (Fig. 11-2*A*). Interference with reabsorption will elevate CSF pressure as shown, for example, by the pressure increase which will occur during lumbar puncture if both internal jugular veins are compressed. Similarly a block of arachnoidal villi by infection or tumor may result in CSF pressures as high as 400 to 500 mm H$_2$O. In an infant, the cranial bones, which are still cartilaginous, may be forced apart by such pressures so that the head may reach enormous size (hydrocephalus) with resultant brain compression, mental retardation and often death.

As mentioned in Chapter 10, a large elevation of CSF pressure will activate the CNS ischemic reflex; arterial pressure then rises linearly to stay above CSF pressure even though cerebral blood flow remains relatively constant (Cushing reflex). The heart rate is usually slowed through baroceptor action; increased arterial pressure in the presence of bradycardia is suggestive of elevated CSF pressure.

Because the brain literally "floats" in CSF, its effective weight *in situ* is reduced from about 1400 g to less than 50 g. This affords cushioning against trauma and reduces the risk of shearing or tearing of the brain tissue from its connections to extracranial tissues as they traverse the various foramina of the skull. Brain injuries may occur upon sudden rotational acceleration of the head, *e.g.,* from a blow to the side of the jaw, or severe linear acceleration which, because of brain inertia, may cause damage at the point opposite the impact (countrecoup).

Blood-Brain Barrier

The capillaries of the brain because of their selective permeability are frequently referred to as a "blood-brain barrier." Most proteins and high molecular weight compounds, dyes, inulin, sucrose, mannitol and catecholamines pass with difficulty or not at all. The relative impermeability to heavy metals and certain antibiotics pose therapeutic problems in the treatment of brain infections. On the other hand, anesthetics (volatile and non-volatile), ethanol, CO_2, O_2, urea and all lipids pass rapidly through brain capillaries. The barrier is partly morphological, *i.e.,* associated with its "tight" endothelial junctions and basement membrane structure (Fig. 11-3). The permeability barrier is in part also due to non-morphological factors, *i.e.,* different diffusion rates and transport mechanisms across these capillaries. While the microstructure of the choroid plexus is unlike that of the brain capillary, the former has a similar permeability barrier so that some investigators refer to a blood-CSF barrier as well as a blood-brain barrier; the similar composition of brain interstitial fluid and CSF would tend to support such a concept.

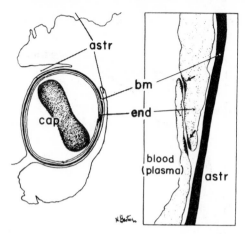

Figure 11-3. Microscopic view of a brain capillary containing an erythrocyte and almost surrounded by the perivascular feet of an astrocyte (*astr*). The capillary membrane consists of endothelial cells (*end*) (with a tight junction) and a continuous basement membrane (*bm*). (From H. D. Patton, J. W. Sundsten, W. E. Crill, and P. D. Swanson, *Introduction to Basic Neurology.* Philadelphia: W. B. Saunders Co., 1976.)

The limited permeability of brain capillaries is diagnostically useful, *e.g.,* in "brain scans" in which a radioactive material such as technetium ([99]TC) adsorbed onto a protein molecule, is injected intravenously; this substance which would ordinarily not penetrate the brain may show up as a darkened area on a gamma screen if the permeability mechanism is damaged by a tumor or infarct.

Measurement of Cerebral Blood Flow (CBF)

The widely used "inert gas" method involves inhalation of a subanesthetic dose of an indicator such as nitrous oxide (N_2O) with periodic measurement of arterial and venous (internal jugular) concentrations until equilibrium which is at about 10 minutes. At this point the arterial and venous N_2O concentrations are equal and that in brain tissue is about equivalent to the 10-minute venous blood sample concentration (Fig. 11-4).

Using the Fick equation (Chapter 7), the cerebral blood flow (CBF) is calculated as follows:

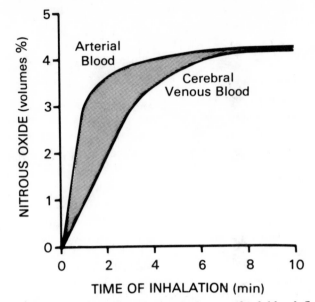

Figure 11-4. Inert gas method for measuring cerebral blood flow (Kety-Schmidt method). N_2O concentrations in arterial and cerebral venous blood while breathing a 15% N_2O gas mixture for 10 minutes. (From S. S. Kety, and C. F. Schmidt, *J. Clin. Invest.* 27:476, 1948.)

$$CBF \text{ (ml/100 g brain tissue/min)} = \frac{100 \times N_2O \text{ uptake}}{(A\text{-}V) \ N_2O \text{ concentration}}$$

so that

$$CBF \text{ (ml/100 g brain tissue/min)} = \frac{100 \times V_{10} \times S}{\int_0^{10} (A\text{-}V) \ dt}$$

in which

$$V_{10} = \text{venous } N_2O \text{ conc at 10 min}$$

and

S = partition coefficient of N_2O in blood and brain which equals one.

Normal Values for CBF in Man. In the normal adult brain, which weighs 1400 to 1500 g, CBF is 50 to 60 ml/100 g brain tissue/min so that total brain flow is about 750 ml/min or 15% of the total cardiac output. The white matter (neuroglia) receives about one half of the average figure but flow to the more vascular gray matter (neurons) is about two times the average.

Characteristics and Control of Cerebral Circulation

Brain is the most vulnerable tissue of the body to ischemia; oxygen deprivation of only seconds may produce unconsciousness and in a few minutes irreversible damage. Fortunately, as many studies have shown, cerebral blood flow tends to remain remarkably constant under most physiological situations. Previously this was attributed to the incompressibility of the cranium and the logical corollary that the combined volume of brain tissue, CSF and intracranial blood must be nearly constant. However, the more likely reason is that the brain has more reflex safeguards to protect its flow than any other organ in the body. These include, *e.g.*, the baroreflexes, the autoregulatory mechanism, the CNS ischemic reflex and (as described below) a specialized flow response to increased Pco_2.

As previously mentioned (Chapter 9), brain vasculature has a well-developed autoregulatory capability which helps to maintain flow relatively constant at variable perfusion pressures; this is also effective in hypertensive patients (Fig. 11-5). Autoregulation in brain as in other tissues, is independent of nervous influences.

Previous data have indicated that brain function, *e.g.*, mental arithmetic, produced only minimal changes in cerebral blood flow; however, newer methods such as radioautography have shown bursts of metabolic activity and flow in very small, localized brain areas coincident with brain activity. For example, simple voluntary contraction of hand muscle is accompanied by a sizable increase in CBF in the localized contralateral hand area of the motor cortex; a light stimulus to the retina will increase blood flow to the superior colliculus and occipital cortex, and during speech, local metabolic activation of the motor speech area of the cortex has been observed. Thus "function mapping" of the brain, using local flow and metabolism as indicators, has now become possible in animals and man and promises to add considerably to our understanding of neural function.

A. Role of CO$_2$ in the Control of Cerebral Blood Flow. Arterial Pco_2 is an important regulator of cerebral flow and Pco_2 alterations exert a profound influence on CBF; hypercapnia causes intense cerebral vasodilation and hypocapnea a marked vasoconstriction (Fig. 11-6*A*). The

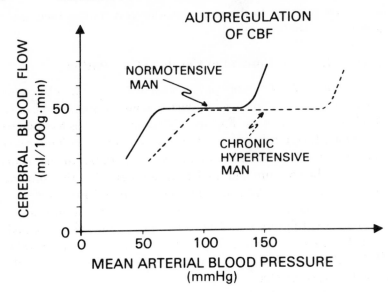

Figure 11-5. Autoregulation of cerebral blood flow in man in normotension and chronic hypertension. In hypertension the autoregulation persists but the curve is shifted to the right. In this study, intracranial pressure, Pco_2 and Po_2 were maintained constant. (From N. A. Lassen, *Peripheral Circulation,* ed. by P. C. Johnson. New York: John Wiley & Sons, 1978.)

CO_2 effect is probably mediated by pH variations in cerebrospinal fluid and apparently serves primarily to maintain the pH of brain tissue; this objective is, in turn, probably associated with the fact that a decreased pH profoundly depresses neuronal activity. Arterial PO_2 changes within the physiological ranges have relatively little effect on CBF (Fig. 11-6*B*). Although some recent studies have indicated the presence of autonomic fibers in the walls of cerebral vessels, the bulk of evidence indicates that they play no significant role in cerebral vascular control.

B. Pathophysiological Aspects of Cerebral Flow. CBF is decreased in surgical anesthesia (as much as 50%) and in cerebral arteriosclerosis. The prevalence of the latter has important clinical implications since cerebral vascular disease is first in frequency among all neurological diseases and furthermore comprises 50% of all neurological hospital admissions to adult wards; the most serious consequence of cerebral arteriosclerosis is "cerebral vascular accident" (CVA or stroke) which

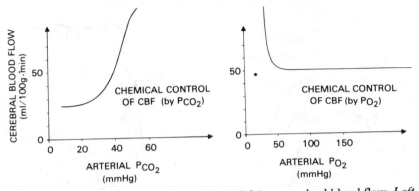

Figure 11-6. Effect of P_{CO_2} (*left*) and P_{O_2} (*right*) on cerebral blood flow. *Left,* note that the steepest part of the P_{CO_2} curve is near 40 mm Hg indicating high sensitivity of CBF to P_{CO_2} at physiological levels. *Right,* at the normal P_{O_2} levels of 80 to 120 mm Hg, the effect on CBF is practically nil. (From N. A. Lassen, *Peripheral Circulation,* ed. by P. A. Johnson. New York: John Wiley & Sons, 1978.)

is due to a thrombus, embolus or rupture of a cerebral artery with resulting infarction of brain tissue. The most common vessel affected is the middle cerebral artery; the clinical results, depending on the branch affected and extent of the infarction, are varying degrees of paralysis and sensory loss over the contralateral half of the body (hemiplegia and hemianesthesia) as well as speech and visual problems. While flow to the infarcted area is diminished, that adjacent to the infarction may have increased flow, presumably due to the accumulation of metabolites at the periphery of the lesion.

CORONARY CIRCULATION

Anatomy

The adult human heart, which has a mass of 250 to 300 g, has three main arteries, the right coronary, supplying the right ventricle and a portion of the posterior left ventricle, and the left anterior descending and circumflex which are the terminal branches of the left coronary and supply primarily the left ventricle (Fig. 11-7). A limited number of small arteries (arterioluminal) run from the main coronary arteries into the ventricles.

The "dominant" supply to the heart is usually determined by that artery which forms the posterior descending; the latter derives from

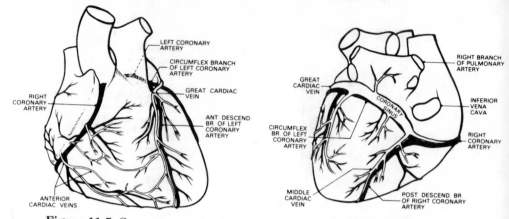

Figure 11-7. Coronary vessels of the human heart. Anterior view (*left*) shows the right coronary artery and anterior descending artery; posterior view (*right*) shows the left circumflex artery and the posterior descending artery. The latter may be formed by the right coronary or left circumflex artery. The anterior cardiac veins from the right ventricle and the coronary sinus, draining primarily the left ventricle, empty into the right atrium.

the left circumflex in 85% of the cases in the dog (left dominance) but in man it is a continuance of the right coronary in about 90% of cases (right dominance). The conventional term 'dominant' refers to the vessel which furnishes the major arterial supply to the inferior wall of the left ventricle and to the AV node; thus the term does not relate to the proportional mass of total myocardium supplied. From a functional standpoint, the anterior descending branch of the left coronary supplies the largest portion of the most important ventricle, *viz.*, the left, and in this sense is the predominant vessel.

The anterior cardiac vein from the right ventricle carries about 15 to 20% of the venous blood and drains into the right atrium. Most of the blood from the left ventricle empties into the great cardiac and other veins and finally into an expanded venous chamber, the coronary sinus; the coronary sinus, which carries 65 to 75% of coronary venous blood, drains into the right atrium. A few small Thebesian veins, carrying about 3 to 5% of the total venous blood, drain directly into the cardiac chambers, mainly the right ventricle (Fig. 11-8).

Capillary and Collateral Circulation

As arteries pass across the surface of the heart, small branches come off at right angles to penetrate the myocardium and end in a rich

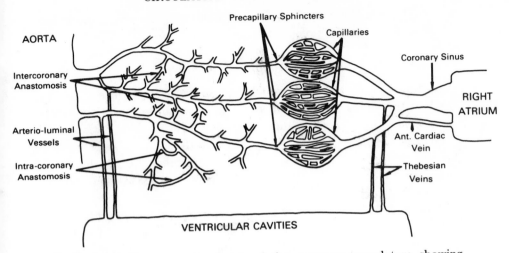

Figure 11-8. Diagrammatic sketch of the coronary vasculature showing arterioluminal vessels, Thebesian veins, collateral arteries and precapillary sphincters.

network of arteries and capillaries. There are precapillary sphincters which play an important role in opening up additional exchange beds during exercise (Fig. 11-8).

Because coronary occlusion is a common clinical entity, the potential for development of collateral vessels becomes very important. Collaterals are anastomotic channels, usually small, pre-existing arterial connections without intervening capillaries. These connections may be between main coronary arteries (intercoronary) or between branches of the same coronary artery (intracoronary) (Fig. 11-8).

The ability to develop collateral vessels varies with different species. In the dog, collateral vessels are located mainly near the epicardium and are relatively plentiful. In man, they are mainly subendocardial and less well developed; in man and in some animal species such as the pig (which has few collaterals), sudden occlusion of a large vessel usually results in a significant infarction (necrosis) with possible cardiac arrest and death. However, with gradual occlusion of even 90% of the lumen of a large vessel (*e.g.,* in the dog), the collaterals open, there is proliferation of the vascular endothelium and smooth muscle cells and within 4 to 8 weeks coronary flow may return almost to the preocclusion level. These vessels apparently develop because of (a) increased wall stress due to heightened pressure gradients, and (b) the action of metabolites resulting from ischemia; the relative importance of these two factors is not yet certain.

Normal Values and General Characteristics

In man, coronary flow is usually measured either by the inert gas method (previously described) involving catheterization of the coronary sinus, or by a "washout" technique following injection of a radioactive agent such as ^{133}Xe or ^{85}Kr into the catheterized coronary artery. Direct measurement with an electromagnetic or ultrasonic flowmeter in an experimental animal permits the recording of phasic flow as shown in Figure 11-9.

The smaller flow in the left coronary during systole (one fifth of the total) is due to the external compression of the artery; the lesser pressures of the right ventricle produce less throttling and permit a proportionately greater systolic flow into the right coronary artery. The normal adult heart has a coronary blood flow of 70 to 80 ml/100 g/min and a total flow of about 250 ml/min, *i.e.*, 4 to 5% of the cardiac output.

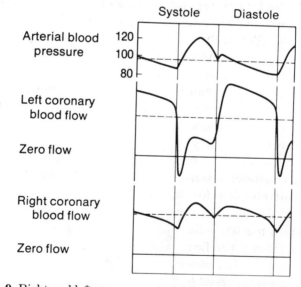

Figure 11-9. Right and left coronary arterial flow during systole and diastole. Note the greater effect of external compression on systolic flow to the left coronary as compared to the right. (From B. Folkow and E. Neil, *Circulation*, London: Oxford University Press, 1971.)

Control of Coronary Circulation

The three main factors influencing flow are (a) *mechanical,* mainly external compression and perfusion pressure, (b) *metabolic* and (c) *neural.*

A. *Mechanical Factors and Coronary Flow.* The compression effect is responsible for 25% of coronary flow resistance at normal heart rates but during tachycardia, when systole occupies an increasing percentage of the cycle, it can account for as much as 55% of vascular resistance. But external compression also affects intramyocardial flow distribution; as the left ventricle contracts, the pressure inside the muscle increases to a level comparable and even higher than the intraventricular pressure (Fig. 11-10). Furthermore, the myocardial pressure is graded, being very low on the epicardial side and at its peak near the endocardium so that subendocardial vessels are compressed the most.

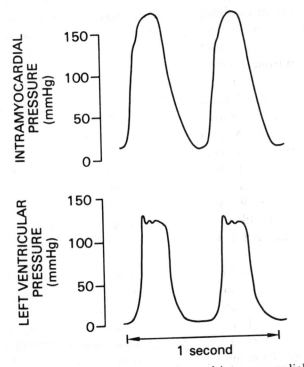

Figure 11-10. Simultaneous intraventricular and intramyocardial pressures from left ventricle of the dog. (From H. Kreuzer, and W. Schoeppe, *Pflügers Arch. Ges. Physiol.* 278:181, 1963.)

As a result subendocardial flow is primarily diastolic. In spite of this, injection of microspheres and other studies indicate that in the normal myocardium, subendocardial and subepicardial flow are about equal. However, when diastolic pressure is low such as in shock, aortic stenosis or coronary occlusion, subendocardial flow decreases dispro-portionately so that this area is more vulnerable to ischemia. This seems to be borne out by the fact that after coronary occlusion, infarcts are more common in the subendocardial area.

Since at normal rates, about 80% of coronary flow occurs in diastole, it follows that aortic diastolic pressure becomes the primary determi-nant of coronary perfusion pressure. Theoretically, coronary flow would, therefore, fluctuate with the diastolic pressure; however, as discussed in Chapter 9, the coronary vessels show a high degree of "autoregulation," i.e., between perfusion pressures of 60 to 180 mm Hg, flow remains relatively constant. Thus the increase in coronary flow which occurs in conditions in which diastolic pressure is elevated is due mainly to the increase in flow accompanying the increased after-load work and increased cardiac metabolism (as described below) rather than from the elevated perfusion pressure.

B. *Cardiac Metabolism and Coronary Flow.* One of the most striking features of myocardial physiology is the close parallelism between metabolic rate and coronary flow; as previously discussed (Chapter 9) a general correlation exists in all tissues. The cause of this metabolic rate-blood flow coupling is not certain. Both increased Pco_2 and reduced pH will increase local flow but unquestionably, hypoxia, i.e., decreased Po_2 is the most potent stimulus of all to coronary flow. The available evidence suggests that either Po_2 itself or a specific metabolite, most likely adenosine, is responsible for the vasodilation. However, other factors such as K^+, osmolality and prostaglandins have been implicated.

C. *Neural Control of Coronary Flow.* The importance of neural factors in coronary control is complicated by their "indirect" effect on the heart itself; this cardiac effect, in turn, then exerts its own influence on coronary flow. For instance, studies on the viable but non-beating heart show that sympathetic stimulation causes both an alpha con-strictor effect (primarily on the epicardial vessels) and a beta dilator effect (mainly endocardial) with a net result of moderate vasodilation in most species. However, in the beating heart, the sympathetic stimulation also causes an increase in rate, myocardial contractility and arterial blood pressure; all three of the latter factors independently increase cardiac work, which is in itself a strong stimulus to coronary flow. Conversely, vagal stimulation by inducing bradycardia, hypotension and decreased cardiac contractility will decrease cardiac metabolism and so produce a marked indirect decrease in coronary flow. It should be noted, however, that carefully designed experiments in which these factors are separately controlled, have suggested that vagal stimulation causes a vasodilation of coronary vessels, a separate and independent effect.

Coronary vessels are also affected by certain cardiovascular reflexes; reports indicate that baroceptor activation *via* stimulation of carotid sinus nerves will result in coronary vasodilation, and stimulation of chemoreceptors apparently causes a tendency toward sympathetic constriction of the coronary arteries. Blood-borne catecholamines will have effects that are similar but of lesser intensity than the corresponding neural stimulation. Epinephrine will directly dilate the coronary vessels but will also greatly stimulate cardiac metabolism to the extent that the increased coronary flow requirements will induce a relative ischemia, which in the coronary patient may be dangerous and even life-threatening.

It is, therefore, evident that because of the close myocardial coupling of flow and metabolism, any increase of cardiac work, which may result from exercise (Fig. 11-11), excitement or the administration of inotropic agents, will induce a corresponding indirect increase in coronary flow.

Oxygen Consumption and Work of the Heart

The "resting" O_2 consumption of the heart is about 8 ml/100 g/min of which about one fourth is for basic maintenance and the remainder for its work of contraction; of the total oxygen consumption, only 35 to 40% is normally due to oxidation of carbohydrates; thus the major cardiac energy (in postabsorptive states) is derived from non-carbohydrate sources, mainly fatty acids. The amino acid contribution is small. As with other tissues, about 95% of the energy is used to form ATP in mitochondria. The main determinants of myocardial oxygen consumption are (a) ventricular wall tension, (b) heart rate, and (c) velocity of myocardial shortening.

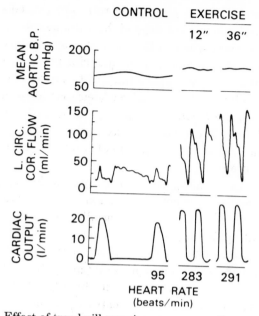

Figure 11-11. Effect of treadmill exercise on coronary flow in the dog. There is a large increase in coronary flow associated with the increased heart rate, blood pressure and cardiac output. (From E. M. Khouri, D. E. Gregg, and C. R. Rayford, *Circ. Res.* 17:427, 1965. By permission of the American Heart Association.)

The main work of the heart is expended by pumping a volume of fluid against a pressure head. For this reason the external cardiac work (for the left ventricle) is usually estimated as the product of the stroke volume ejected and the mean aortic pressure during systole (stroke work). The "pressure work" may also be approximated as the product of the cardiac output and the mean arterial pressure. Since the mean pulmonary arterial pressure is about one sixth that of the aorta and the output of the right ventricle the same as the left, the work done per minute by the right ventricle is about one sixth that of the left.

But in addition to the potential energy in the form of pressure-volume work, kinetic energy is also generated because of the velocity imparted to the blood. Although at rest only about 2 to 4% of the useful work of the heart is in the form of kinetic energy, this fraction may increase to 20 or 25% in exercise.

Because cardiac pressure work is more demanding of oxygen than "flow work," Sarnoff and associates suggested that myocardial O_2 consumption ($M\dot{V}O_2$) might be indirectly estimated by the "tension-time index" (TTI) which is the product of the left ventricular pressure/time integral and the heart rate. In a condition such as aortic stenosis (Chapter 3), intraventricular pressure (and thus TTI and cardiac work) will be much elevated; this increased work requirement prevails in the face of a lessened aortic pressure available for coronary perfusion.

Recent studies by Bruce and others on exercise in normal subjects and cardiac patients have indicated that certain indices such as the product of systolic pressure and heart rate (pressure-pulse or double product) or the systolic pressure-heart rate-systolic ejection time product (triple product) are highly correlated with myocardial oxygen consumption ($M\dot{V}O_2$). The double product at maximal exercise can thus provide a reasonable non-invasive estimate of the limit of left ventricular capability. It should be pointed out, however, that TTI and double product estimations of coronary $M\dot{V}O_2$ do not take into account the metabolic effect of increase in wall tension which occurs in dilated hearts (LaPlace's law, Chapter 1) or the alteration in contraction velocity which also has a metabolic effect as mentioned above.

Efficiency of the Heart

Mechanical efficiency is usually estimated as external work done divided by energy consumed. The work may be calculated as described above and the energy by conversion of O_2 consumption (1 ml O_2 liberates 2.06 kg m of energy). The efficiency of the myocardium is ordinarily about 5 to 15% although this may be considerably increased in exercise in which the cardiac output or flow component increases disproportionately to the pressure component. The remaining 85 to 95% of the energy produced is in the form of heat; because of the metabolism-stimulating and flow-stimulating effects of temperature itself, physical work capacity is importantly influenced by the ability of the body to maintain minimum temperature. The increased blood flow to skin which occurs in order to dissipate the excess heat, adds to cardiac work demands and, therefore, to coronary flow requirements; this may be a limiting factor in the work capacity of cardiac patients.

It is undoubtedly evident from the foregoing that the coronary circulation presents more complexities and investigative difficulties than any other regional circulation. Among such problems are the vagaries of the arterial and venous anatomy and the difficulty of access for circulatory measurements on a moving organ. While possible relevance to intact man is a perpetual problem in experimental physiology, the applicability to man of coronary studies in animals must be weighed with special care because of significant differences among species, the effects of anesthesia, and finally, the indirect effects of any intervention such as a drug on the heart itself.

CUTANEOUS CIRCULATION

The main function of skin circulation is to maintain temperature balance by providing (a) insulation against cold and (b) efficient heat transfer between the body core and the periphery. This heat-regulating mechanism, aided by sweat production and evaporative cooling, is much better adapted to protect against over-heating than against excessive cold.

Anatomy of Skin Vasculature

Skin has a variable thickness, generally 1 to 3 mm, a surface area in the 70-kg adult of 1.7 to 1.8 m^2 and an aggregate mass of 2 to 2.5 kg, about 4% of the total body weight. From a functional standpoint, the vasculature is of two general types: the first is an extensive, superficial arteriolar-capillary-venular network of the usual architecture with an extensive, slow-flowing subcutaneous venous plexus; this general structure prevails over most of the body with particularly rich networks in the forearm, legs and thighs. The second vascular arrangement, which is found in palms of the hands, soles of the feet and in the face (especially the ears, nose and lips), is similar to the above but has, in addition a large number of unique arteriovenous anastamoses (AVAs); skin in these areas is studded with numerous such capillary bypasses which consist of coiled arterial vessels about 50 μm in diameter with thick muscular walls, well supplied with sympathetic nerve fibers. These vessels do not have capillary exchange surfaces and by virtue of their unusual vascularity are capable of large heat exchanges (Fig. 11-12).

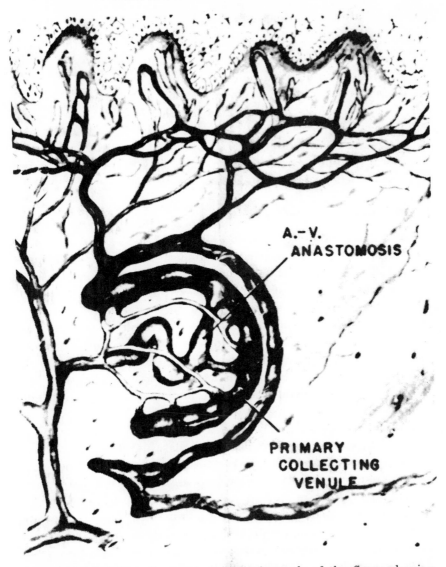

Figure 11-12. Schematic drawing of blood vessels of the finger showing superficial plexus and an AV anastamosis which connects directly to a venule of the subcutaneous plexus. When dilated, the AVAs are capable of huge increases in flow. (From A. C. Hseih, in *The Peripheral Circulations,* ed. by R. Zelis. New York: Grune & Stratton Inc., 1975.)

Normal Values and Response Range

Skin blood flow is commonly determined in man with the venous occlusion plethysmograph (Chapter 4). Such studies have shown that this tissue is capable of extreme flow ranges; under maximum heat stimulation, hand skin flow can increase about 30-fold from the normal values of 3 to 5 ml/100 g tissue/min and with cold application of 15°C, 10-fold decreases to 0.3 to 0.5 ml/100 g/min. With further cooling, *e.g.*, to 10°C, there follows, however, a cold-induced vasodilation, a protective, local, non-neurogenic reaction, sometimes called the "hunting response." Its mechanism is unknown.

Control of Skin Blood Vessels

While there are direct blood flow effects of heat and cold on skin, as described above, by far the main mechanism is an "indirect" sympathetic reflex response. This is due to a stimulation of heat-sensitive thermoreceptors in the skin and in the hypothalamus (*via* warmed blood) which markedly vasodilate resistance vessels (*i.e.*, arterioles and AVAs) as well as capacitance vessels. The result is a large increase in both arterial flow and in the slow-velocity, subcutaneous venous flow, the latter being especially well-adapted to transfer heat to the environment. Vasodilation in the hands, feet and face is "passive," *i.e.*, due to reduction in sympathetic tone, but in other areas is mainly "active" (Fig. 11-13).

This active vasodilation is carried out by arterioles, but not by AVAs; some investigators have proposed that this dilation mechanism is similar to that prevailing in certain glandular tissues and sweat glands and that it involves the local release of an enzyme which acts on a globulin substrate to liberate bradykinin, a potent vasodilator.

The reflex response to cold, while less marked, is significant and includes not only reduction of arterial flow but also venoconstriction, with a resultant decrease in subcutaneous venous volume and an increase in velocity of venous blood flow, a distinct advantage in minimizing heat loss. During severe and prolonged cold, the direct effects, added to the indirect reflex effects, may so reduce skin flow that it is almost immeasurable, with the distinct risk of frostbite and severe tissue damage. Frostbite was previously discussed in Chapter 2 under blood viscosity.

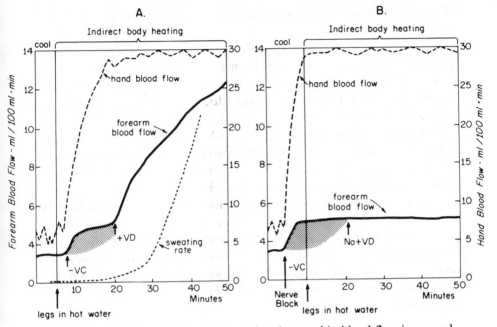

Figure 11-13. Reflex effects of indirect heating on skin blood flow in normal hand and forearm i.e. changes in finger and forearm blood flow when legs were put in hot H_2O. *A,* Vasodilation in the hand is mediated only by release of tonic sympathetic vasoconstrictor tone (−VC); this "passive" vasodilation accounts, however, for only a small part of the blood flow in the forearm (−VC to +VD). The remainder, as well as the sweating, is due to active sympathetic vasodilation and can be prevented by sympathetic blockade, *B;* note in *B* the abrupt increase in hand (skin) blood flow after nerve block illustrating the neurogenic control of skin blood flow. However (in B) the nerve block prevented the increase in forearm blood flow. (From J. T. Shepherd, *Physiology of Circulation in Human Limbs in Health and Disease.* Philadelphia: W. B. Saunders Co., 1963.)

Pathophysiological Responses

Inflammation of the skin or pressure on the skin surface induces a vascular reaction depending on the intensity of the stimulus. After light stroking there is pallor and after a heavier stroking a red line due to venular dilation. Upon repeated or heavier pressure, the reddening or "flare" will occur and spread because of arteriolar involvement; with still greater trauma, wheals will result. This sequence has been called the "triple response" and is ascribed to the local production and spread of histamine; it involves a local vascular mechanism and is thought to be an axon reflex.

Blood vessels of skin are unusually sensitive to central nervous and hormonal influences. Fear may be marked by vasoconstriction and pallor; cold sweats may occur due to nervous tension, and blushing will follow certain emotional stimuli, although the latter response is reportedly becoming extinct in Western civilization.

The unusual sensitivity of skin vessels to nervous and hormonal influences makes this tissue vulnerable to certain vasospastic disorders of the extremities. *Raynaud's disease,* a chronic condition of this type, affects the hands and occurs particularly in women in colder climates. It is characterized by frequent vasospasms and blanching of the fingers of both hands followed by vasodilation, ischemic pain and in some cases eventual tissue necrosis. The condition is thought to be an exaggerated vasoconstrictor response to continued sympathoadrenal stimulation associated with nervous tension. Bilateral upper thoracic sympathectomy is sometimes helpful but usually does not afford lasting relief.

CIRCULATION IN SKELETAL MUSCLE

The primary function of these vessels is to serve the metabolic needs of skeletal muscle, needs which can increase as much as 100-fold over the resting level. Because of the great muscle mass, a secondary role is to provide a reserve of vascular resistance for certain emergencies such as circulatory shock. Muscle circulation has two quite different mechanisms to discharge these two different functions, *i.e.,* a local metabolic and central neural control system.

General Flow Characteristics and Normal Values

As mentioned in Chapter 9, at rest 20 to 25% of the cardiac output supplies the skeletal muscles with about 4 to 6 ml of flow per 100 g/min; however, at maximal exercise almost 90% of the cardiac output may be diverted to the working muscles (Chapter 12). Rapid, phasic (white) fiber units, which comprise 80 to 85% of the muscle mass, may upon contraction increase their flow 10-fold from a resting level of 2 to 4 ml/100 g/min while the slow, tonic (red) fibers, may experience a 4-fold increase from somewhat higher resting values of 20 to 30 ml/100 g/min. In experimental animals such flow determinations are usually made by direct flowmetering of the arteries and in man by means of venous occlusion plethysmography (Chapter 4).

Muscle arterioles have a high resting tone, most of which is inherent in the vascular muscle itself (myogenic tone) and the remainder due to a tonic sympathetic vasoconstrictor outflow with a frequency of about one impulse/sec. An increase in the stimulation frequency to 4 to 5 imp/sec produces about a 70% reduction in flow but has a lesser effect on exercising muscle (Fig. 11-14).

Local (Metabolic) Control of Muscle Circulation during Exercise

At rest the neural factors are primary but during muscle contraction the local metabolism becomes practically the exclusive regulator of the

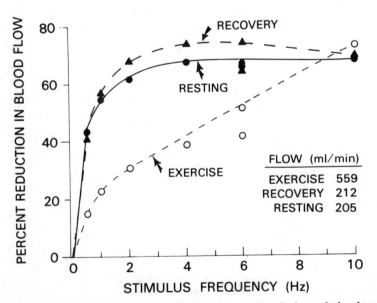

Figure 11-14. Effect of frequency of electrical stimulation of the lumbar sympathetic chain on limb blood flow in the dog. At rest there was marked flow reduction with increase in frequency. During exercise the stimulation was less effective because the bed was under metabolic control. (From D. E. Donald, D. J. Rowlands, and D. A. Ferguson, *Circ. Res.* 26:185, 1970. By permission of the American Heart Association.)

muscle flow; skeletal muscle has well developed autoregulatory and reactive hyperemic properties, a further manifestation of the link between metabolism and flow in this bed. During rhythmic exercise, flow is intermittent because of the mechanical compression effect on the vasculature. Flow interference begins at about 30% of maximum tension with complete stoppage at about the 70% level; this deprives the fiber of oxygen at its time of greatest need although the myoglobin of red muscles provides some assistance through its oxygen "accumulator" and release action. On the venous side, this intermittent compression of veins in conjunction with venous valves, produces a strong phasic milking action (Chapter 4); the resultant lowering of net venous pressure is thought to play an important role in increasing perfusion through lower extremity muscles during exercise such as running.

As with other vascular beds, considerable effort has been directed to the study of the possible mechanism of the hyperemia during increased metabolism. A number of vasodilator substances have been proposed, most prominently Po_2, H^+, K^+ and adenosine; as yet there is no agreement on any one agent.

Some investigators believe that local hyperosmolality may be a factor, at least in initiating the hyperemic response. With exercise there is known to be a metabolic breakdown within the muscle cell of many large molecules into smaller ones, increasing osmolality and causing transfer of water into the cell; this is probably responsible for the 10 to 15% decrease in plasma volume which is usual after exercise.

Central (Neural) Control of Muscle Circulation

Sympathetic vasoconstriction is the primary circulatory control mechanism of skeletal muscle in non-exercise situations (Fig. 11-14). Vasodilation can be brought about either passively by decreased stimulation of vasoconstrictors (which is the most common mechanism) or actively *via* sympathetic cholinergic or beta adrenergic vasodilators. Cholinergic vasodilation mainly results from cerebral activity such as mental effort or emotion; it is thought that these descending impulses from the higher centers may bypass the medullary cardiovascular centers.

Skeletal muscle vessels are also important participants in reflex response. Increased stimulation of arterial baroceptors and certain cardiopulmonary receptors will result in decreased sympathetic tone and passive vasodilation of skeletal muscle resistance vessels; it is also thought that some active vasodilation also occurs, at least initially. Conversely, decreased stimulation of arterial and cardiopulmonary receptors will result in reflex sympathetic vasoconstriction in skeletal muscle (Fig. 11-15).

Stimulation of aortic and carotid body chemoreceptors, *e.g.,* during hypoxia or shock, will also induce reflex vasoconstriction in skeletal muscle. If, however, a vasodilation stimulus is imposed on a bed previously vasoconstricted, *e.g.,* by hemorrhage or hypoxia, such sudden inhibition—accompanied as it sometimes is by vagal bradycardia—can lower peripheral resistance sharply and result in fainting (Chapter 13).

It should also be mentioned that muscle veins, in sharp contrast to

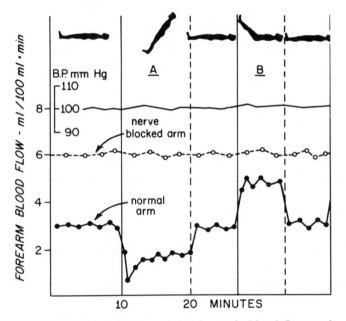

Figure 11-15. Response of forearm skeletal muscle blood flow to decreased (*A*) and increased (*B*) cardiopulmonary receptor stimulation due to intrathoracic blood volume changes. These changes were produced by head-up tilt and leg raising, respectively. Sympathetic blockade in the control arm prevented the flow changes. Arterial baroceptors were not involved since arterial pressure did not change. (From J. T. Shepherd, *Physiology of the Circulation in Human Limbs in Health and Disease.* Philadelphia: W. B. Saunders Co., 1963.)

splanchnic and cutaneous veins, are practically devoid of adrenergic nerve endings in their walls and as a consequence these veins react little if at all to sympathetic vasomotor constriction and so do not serve a significant reservoir function.

Neurohormonal Effects

Under certain circumstances, catecholamines may influence muscle vasculature. As described in Chapter 9 the arterioles of skeletal muscle contain sympathetic alpha, beta and cholinergic receptors so that the result of sympathetic stimulation is usually a balance between two or more effects. Norepinephrine (NE) injection has a small beta dilator, but a much stronger alpha constrictor action; a moderate intravenous dose of NE in the intact organism will, therefore, raise the blood pressure and thereby activate the arterial baroceptors, producing a subsequent reflex vasodilation and corrective fall in pressure. Epinephrine usually induces a marked but transitory beta dilator action which is enhanced if its secondary effect, an alpha constrictor action, is blocked (Chapter 9).

PULMONARY CIRCULATION

Anatomy

The pulmonary and systemic circuits are in series and in the normal resting adult, each ventricle has an output of about 70 ml/kg/min or 5 L/min. The pulmonary circulation, with only one tenth the capacity of the systemic, must, in the same time period, accommodate the same ejected volume. The pulmonary vessels, which are much shorter, accommodate this volume without excessive pressure fluctuations because of thinner walls and greater compliance. The pulmonary capillaries form a very thin, rich, vascular network around the alveoli which facilitates blood-gas exchange.

Pressure and Flow in the Pulmonary Vessels

The mean pressures in the right ventricle and pulmonary artery are about one sixth as great as those of the left ventricle and aorta (Fig. 11-16). Since the total flows are equal, the pulmonary vascular resistance is only one sixth that of the systemic (Fig. 11-16). However, the pressure waves, flow patterns and cardiac valvular movements of these

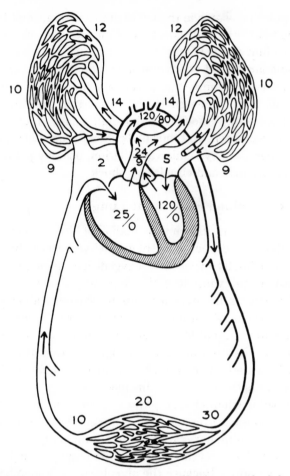

Figure 11-16. Representative pressures (mm Hg) in normal adult pulmonary and systemic circulations. (Reproduced with permission from J. H. Comroe, *Physiology of Respiration,* 2nd ed, Copyright © 1974 by Year Book Medical Publishers, Inc., Chicago.)

two circuits are quite similar. The normal mean pressure in the pulmonary artery is about 15 mm Hg, in the capillaries about 10 mm Hg and in the pulmonary veins and left atrium about 5 mm Hg. Thus the pulmonary arterial-capillary gradient is about equal to the pulmonary capillary-venous gradient (about 5 mm Hg) indicating that these two segments contribute about equally to pulmonary vascular resistance, a very different situation than in the systemic circuit. The mean and pulse pressures in the left atrium are somewhat higher than those of the right (Fig. 11-16) because of the more forceful contractions of the left atrium and ventricle.

The pulmonary blood volume, usually about 450 ml or 10% of the total, often serves an important secondary function as a reserve vascular volume. It is increased in the supine position, in exercise or generalized systemic vasoconstriction, left heart failure and mitral stenosis. It is decreased, and thus diverted into the general circulation, in case of generalized systemic vasodilation, positive pressure breathing, the erect posture and circulatory shock.

Distribution of Blood Flow in the Lung

In order to carry out its primary mission of blood-gas exchange, it is necessary that the oxygen-poor blood delivered *via* the pulmonary arteries be maximally exposed to oxygen-rich air of the alveoli, *i.e.,* that perfusion and ventilation be kept in balance. An imbalance between these two is, however, a common occurrence and is responsible for most gas exchange problems in pulmonary disease. One factor contributing to the ventilation-perfusion imbalance is the effect of posture on flow distribution; in the upright position, there is minimal flow to the lung apex and a progressively increasing rate of flow toward the base. What is the reason for this inequality?

As described in Chapter 4, respiratory excursions induce fluctuating negative intrathoracic pressures; these pressures are exerted, however, mainly on the pulmonary arterial and pulmonary venous vessels. Pulmonary capillaries on the other hand are more strongly influenced by alveolar pressures. Because the alveolocapillary membrane is thin and pliant, the effective extravascular capillary pressure normally approximates the alveolar pressure (P_A) rather than the more negative intrathoracic pressure. But in the upright position there may be a hydrostatic pressure difference of 30 cm H_2O (23 mm Hg) between the apex and base of the lung. Since the normal pulmonary artery pressure is only about 20 cm H_2O, this hydrostatic pressure difference has important pulmonary hemodynamic consequences.

Since at the lung apex, *i.e.,* above the heart, the pulmonary intracapillary pressure may be lower than alveolar pressure, some of the capillaries may collapse and flow at the apex will be less than that at the base (Fig. 11-17, zone 1). However, at the base (zone 3, Fig. 11-17),

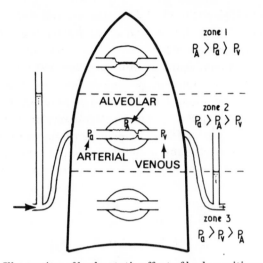

zone 1
$P_A > P_a > P_v$

ALVEOLAR

zone 2
$P_a > P_A > P_v$

ARTERIAL VENOUS

zone 3
$P_a > P_v > P_A$

Figure 11-17. Illustration of hydrostatic effect of body position on pulmonary capillary flow. In zone 1 above heart level, the extramural pulmonary alveolar pressure (P_A) may be greater than the pulmonary capillary pressure and some capillaries may collapse. In zone 2, flow may be intermittent; in zone 3 below the heart, with increased hydrostatic pressure, the capillaries distend and flow is increased. (From J. B. West, C. T. Dollery, and A. Naimark, *J. Appl. Physiol.* 19:713, 1964.)

the added hydrostatic pressure increases the capillary transmural pressure well beyond the alveolar pressure so the vessels will not only remain patent but are distended and flow will be increased. In this situation it is seen that flow depends, not only on the usual longitudinal driving pressure gradient but also on the transmural pressure gradient which must be positive in order to prevent collapse.

In the upright subject the ventilation-perfusion ratio is greater than one at the apex and decreases to values below one at the base. In the normal individual this is not a serious handicap to gas exchange; however, if there is a pathological deficiency of either ventilation or perfusion, this potential handicap can be exaggerated and present a serious threat to possible gas exchange.

Control of Pulmonary Vessels

The pulmonary circulation acts mainly as a passive, compliant, vascular bed, adapting to the demands of the circulation at large. Most studies indicate that although the vessels are well supplied with vagal and sympathetic fibers, these apparently have little functional role. Pulmonary vessels will, however, constrict strongly under the influence of hypoxia. This is a regional phenomenon which occurs in the area of the hypoxia and may be due to local release of a vasoconstrictor substance. It should be noted that this pulmonary vasoconstrictor response is directly opposite to the usual vasodilator effect of hypoxia in all other circulatory beds. The hypoxic vasoconstriction is reinforced by similar vasoconstrictor action of decreased pH which often coexists. Hypoxic vasoconstriction serves a useful purpose in diverting the flow from poorly ventilated regions to other lung areas with more abundant oxygen, thus improving the overall gas exchange. Hypoxic vasoconstriction, which may occur at altitude or in patients with chronic obstructive pulmonary disease, can—if prolonged—lead to pulmonary hypertension.

Drugs which constrict pulmonary vessels include norepinephrine, serotonin, histamine and a number of the prostaglandins. Isoproterenol and acetylcholine are vasodilators.

Pulmonary Capillary Dynamics and Edema

The combination of a plasma osmotic pressure of about 28 mm Hg and a low pulmonary capillary hydrostatic pressure of 10 mm Hg results in a rather unusual net inward force of about 18 mm Hg. This factor coupled with a rather "tight" capillary endothelium helps to maintain narrow interstitial spaces between the capillary and alveolar surfaces which in turn expedites gaseous diffusion. This negative pressure gradient represents a safety factor reducing the chances of interstitial fluid accumulation; pulmonary edema will, for example, usually not occur in experimental animals until left atrial pressure exceeds 20 mm Hg. In case of severe left ventricular failure or mitral stenosis, however, left atrial pressure and volume will steadily increase with an eventual damming effect and an increase in pulmonary venous and capillary pressures; interstitial edema will then develop and if the process continues, fluid will also accumulate in the alveoli resulting in progressive interference with oxygenation, shortness of breath and difficulty in breathing, i.e., dyspnea (Chapter 14).

REFERENCES

General

ABBOUD, F. M., D. D. HEISTAD, A. L. MARK, AND P. G. SCHMID: Reflex control of the peripheral circulation. *Prog. Cardiovasc. Dis.* 18(No.5):371, 1976.

FOLKOW, B., AND E. NEIL: *Circulation.* New York: Oxford University Press, 1971.

HADDY, F. J., AND J. B. SCOTT: Metabolically linked vasoactive chemicals in local regulation of blood flow. *Physiol. Rev.* 48:688, 1968.

JOHNSON, P. C.: *Peripheral Circulation.* New York: John Wiley & Sons, 1978.

KORNER, P. I.: Control of blood flow to special vascular areas: Brain, kidney, muscle, skin, liver and intestine. In *Cardiovascular Physiology,* MTP International Review of Science, ed. by A. C. Guyton and C. E. Jones. Baltimore: University Park Press, 1974.

ROWELL, L. B.: Human cardiovascular adjustment to exercise and thermal stress. *Physiol. Rev.* 54(1):75, 1974.

SHEPHERD, J. T.: *Physiology of the Circulation in Human Limb in Health and Disease.* Philadelphia: W. B. Saunders Co., 1963.

SPARKS, H. V.: Skin and muscle. In *Peripheral Circulation,* ed. by P. C. Johnson. New York: John Wiley & Sons, 1978.

ZELIS, R.: *The Peripheral Circulations.* New York: Grune & Stratton Inc., 1975.

Cerebral Circulation

FISHER, C. M., J. P. MOHR, AND R. D. ADAMS: Cerebrovascular diseases. In *Principles of Internal Medicine,* 7th ed., ed. by M. M. Wintrobe, p. 1743. New York: McGraw-Hill Book Co., 1974.

KETY, S. S., AND C. F. SCHMIDT: The nitrous oxide method for the determination of cerebral blood flow in man: Theory, procedure and normal values. *J. Clin. Invest.* 27:476, 1948.

LASSEN, N. A.: Brain. In *Peripheral Circulation,* ed. by P. C. Johnson. New York: John Wiley & Sons, 1978.

PATTON, H. D., J. W. SUNDSTEN, W. E. CRILL, AND P. D. SWANSON: *Introduction to Basic Neurology.* Philadelphia: W. B. Saunders Co., 1976.

Coronary Circulation

AMSTERDAM, E. A., J. L. HUGHES, A. N. DeMARIA, R. ZELIS, AND D. T. MASON: Indirect assessment of myocardial oxygen consumption in the evaluation of mechanisms and therapy of angina pectoris. *Am. J. Cardiol.* 33:737, 1974.

BERNE, R. M.: Regulation of coronary blood flow. *Physiol. Rev.* 204:317, 1963.

BRAUNWALD, E., J. ROSS, AND E. H. SONNENBLICK: Regulation of coronary blood flow. In *Mechanisms of Contraction of the Normal and Failing Heart.* Boston: Little, Brown and Co., 1976.

BRUCE, R. A., L. D. FISHER, M. N. COOPER, AND G. O. GEY: Separation of effects of cardiovascular disease and age on ventricular function with maximal exercise. *Am. J. Cardiol.* 34:757, 1974.

FEIGL, E. O.: The coronary circulation. In *Physiology and Biophysics,* ed. by T. C. Ruch and H. D. Patton. Philadelphia: W. B. Saunders Co., 1974.

KITAMURA, K., C. R. JORGENSEN, F. L. GOBEL, H. L. TAYLOR, AND Y. WANG: Hemodynamic correlates of myocardial oxygen consumption during upright exercise. *J. Appl. Physiol.* 32:516, 1972.

JAMES, T. N.: *Anatomy of the Coronary Arteries.* New York: Hoeber Medical Division, Harper & Row, Publishers, Inc., 1961.

RUBIO, R., AND R. M. BERNE: Myocardium. In *Peripheral Circulation,* ed. by P. C. Johnson. New York: John Wiley & Sons, 1978.

SARNOFF, S. J., E. BRAUNWALD, G. H. WELCH, R. B. CASE, W. N. STAINSBY, AND R. MACRUZ: Hemodynamic determinants of oxygen consumption of the heart with special reference to the tension-time-index. *Am. J. Physiol.* 192: 148, 1958.

Cutaneous Circulation

COOPER, K. E., R. H. JOHNSON, AND J. M. K. SPALDING: The effects of central body and trunk skin temperatures on reflex vasodilation in the hand. *J. Physiol.* 174:46, 1964.

GREENFIELD, A. D. M.: The circulation through the skin. In *Handbook of Physiology,* Section 2; *Circulation,* vol. II, ed. by W. F. Hamilton and P. Dow. Washington, D.C., American Physiological Society, 1963.

ROWELL, L. B., J. A. MURRAY, G. L. BRENGELMANN, AND K. K. KRANING: Human cardiovascular adjustment to rapid changes in skin temperature during exercise. *Circ. Res.* 24:711, 1969.

Skeletal Muscle Circulation

GREENFIELD, A. D. M., R. J. WHITNEY, AND J. F. MOWBRAY: Methods for investigation of peripheral blood flow. *Br. Med. Bull.* 19:101, 1963.

MELLANDER, S., AND B. JOHANSSON: Control of resistance, exchange and capacitance functions in peripheral circulation. *Pharmacol. Rev.* 20:117, 1968.

Pulmonary Circulation

CUMMING, G.: The pulmonary circulation. In *Cardiovascular Physiology,* MTP International Review of Science, ed. by A. C. Guyton and C. P. Jones. Baltimore: University Park Press, 1974.

GREEN, J. F.: The pulmonary circulation. In *The Peripheral Circulations,* ed. by R. Zelis. New York: Grune & Stratton Inc., 1975.

WEST, J. B.: *Respiratory Physiology,* 2nd ed. Baltimore: Williams & Wilkins Co., 1979.

chapter 12

Physiology of Exercise and the Effect of Aging

Physical exercise is one of the most physiologically demanding activities engaged in by man. Even upon anticipation, there occurs a strong sympathoadrenal activation, particularly if there is an emotional element involved. When muscular activity begins, there rapidly follows a complex and highly integrated series of neuromuscular, respiratory, circulatory and metabolic events which permit the transformation of chemical energy into muscular work. During recovery there is an orderly payback of the oxygen debt which has been accumulated.

While many systems are involved, emphasis in this chapter is on cardiovascular response to exercise (both isotonic and isometric), on physical training and on exercise stress testing. Because of the increased interest in the effects of aging on cardiovascular performance, we have also incorporated a brief account of some recent studies in this field.

DYNAMIC (ISOTONIC) EXERCISE

Dynamic exercise refers to repeated voluntary muscle movements in which there is alternate contraction and relaxation of the muscle, as distinct from isometric (static) exercise, in which the muscle is kept in a state of continued contraction.

General Circulatory Response to Exercise

With the rapid increase in energy requirements, equally rapid circulatory adjustments are essential in order to meet the increased need for O_2 and nutrients by the exercising muscle. Also important is the need to remove the end products of metabolism such as CO_2 and lactic acid and to dissipate the excess heat produced by the reactions. The emphasis in this section is on how the circulatory system meets these increased demands.

Any muscle work that requires an energy expenditure greater than can be supplied by the ongoing oxidative processes is termed anaerobic; this situation prevails at the onset and during the intensive stages of exercise. The lactic acid and other metabolites that accumulate during anaerobic exercise represent an oxygen debt that must be repaid during recovery in order to restore the metabolic system.

The increase in oxygen consumption ($\dot{V}_{O_2}$) during exercise is directly proportional to the work performed up to maximal work capacity ($\dot{V}_{O_2max}$). The increased oxygen demand is met through an increase both in cardiac output and in O_2 extraction from the blood. With a typical 4- to 5-fold increase in CO and a 2- to 3-fold increase in A-V O_2 difference, $\dot{V}_{O_2}$ can be increased 8- to 15-fold. Exceptional athletes may achieve values of $\dot{V}_{O_2max}$ between 5 and 6 liters per minute, a 20-fold increase over resting levels.

How is this extraordinary shift in body metabolism brought about? Mainly through the greatly increased and superbly coordinated activity of almost all systems of the body, *i.e.*, neuromuscular, respiratory, cardiovascular, metabolic and hormonal.

In the circulatory system of normal individuals, there is an approximately linear relationship between total oxygen consumption ($\dot{V}_{O_2}$) and heart rate (HR), cardiac output (CO) and minute ventilation ($\dot{V}_E$) (Fig. 12-1). At or near maximal working capacity ($\dot{V}_{O_2max}$), CO and HR tend to plateau whereas $\dot{V}_E$ tends to rise even more rapidly.

The increased HR is due partly to sympathetic hyperactivity and partly to reduced vagal tone. The maximal heart rate (HR_{max}), *i.e.*, that rate achieved at $\dot{V}_{O_2max}$, is an important limiting factor in cardiovascular performance and is age-dependent. Although there is considerable individual variability in HR_{max} at any age, it can be approximated by the formula, $HR_{max} = 220 - $ age (in years).

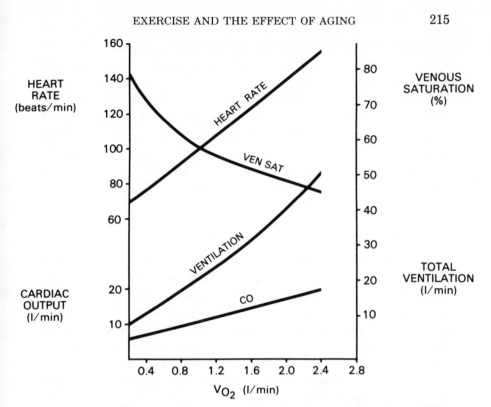

Figure 12-1. Effect of progressive exercise on heart rate, cardiac output (CO), ventilation and venous HbO$_2$ saturation. (From Starling and Evans, *Principles of Human Physiology*, 14th ed. Philadelphia: Lea & Febiger, 1968.)

There is an increase in stroke volume with exercise. Some of the past controversy regarding stroke volume response to exercise is now known to have been due to postural effects. In upright exercise, stroke volume is initially smaller but increases progressively at increasing work levels until about 40% of $\dot{V}_{O_2max}$, at which point it reaches its maximal value and plateaus. In supine exercise, because of increased filling pressure, stroke volume is initially greater (than in the upright) and with increasing exercise is maintained nearly constant, so that the CO increase in the supine is achieved mainly through increase in HR. Final CO levels are very similar at equivalent work loads in the two positions.

The increased stroke volume is due to both an increased diastolic filling with a resultant increased force of ventricular contraction (Starling effect) and increased myocardial contractility due to sympathetic stimulation with a resultant increase in velocity of myocardial contraction (positive inotropic effect).

There is a pronounced rise in systolic pressure (SP), the increase being in approximate proportion to the intensity of the exercise; SP reaches levels of about 170 to 200 mm Hg at $\dot{V}o_{2max}$. In spite of the great increase in cardiac output (4- to 5-fold), diastolic pressure is changed very little because of the considerable decline in peripheral resistance. The result is an increase in pulse pressure which parallels the rise in systolic pressure.

Distribution of Blood Flow in Exercise

A rise in blood flow to the exercising muscles is brought about through both an increase and a redistribution of CO. At rest, only about 15 to 20% of CO is distributed to skeletal muscle in contrast to 85 or 90% during maximal exercise. This represents a 15- to 20-fold increase in flow to the skeletal muscles and a 3- to 4-fold increase to the myocardium (Fig. 12-2). While both total and fractional flow to exercising skeletal muscle is increasing greatly, brain blood flow stays about the same; however, there is a marked decrease in flow to most other regions of the body (Fig. 12-2).

The redistribution of blood flow in exercise is initiated by the anticipatory sympathetic cholinergic vasodilation to skeletal muscle and strongly reinforced by (a) sympathetic vasoconstriction to non-exercising tissues such as kidney, splanchnic area and non-exercising muscle, and (b) metabolic hyperemia in the exercising muscle. This redistribution is highly important in conserving blood flow and therefore oxygen for active muscle (Fig. 12-3).

Thermoregulatory adjustments are essential in any exercise which lasts more than a few minutes since 80% of the total energy produced is thermal and must be carried to the skin surface to be dissipated. In moderate exercise, skin blood flow usually increases 3- to 4-fold. In severe exercise a constrictor tendency manifests itself and flow returns toward baseline levels apparently in an effort toward maximum conservation of flow for skeletal muscle exchange (Fig. 12-2). The hypothalamus is the essential integrator for both the vasomotor and the thermoregulatory changes.

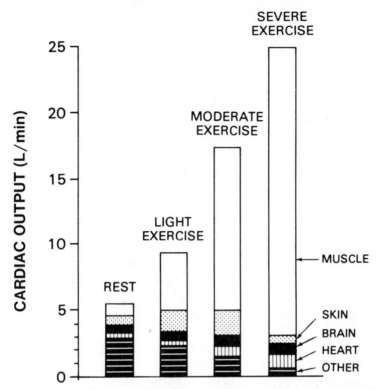

Figure 12-2. Distribution of blood flow with increasing levels of exercise in man. In severe exercise there is about a 20-fold increase in skeletal muscle flow and a 4-fold increase in coronary flow with little change in brain blood flow and a marked decrease to almost all remaining tissues. (From Starling and Evans, *Principles of Human Physiology*, Philadelphia: Lea & Febiger, 1968.)

Systemic Response to Exercise

In the normal individual, the arterial Po_2 is unchanged even in severe exercise, indicating that pulmonary ventilation is not the limiting factor. There is, however, a progressive decrease in venous O_2 saturation (Fig. 12-1) and, therefore, an increasing A-V O_2 difference, indicating a heightened extraction of O_2 by the tissues. The O_2 extraction, which is greater in cardiac patients at similar work loads, is sometimes used as an index of decreased cardiac output in cardiac decompensation.

Important changes occur in blood chemistry. Because of the intense

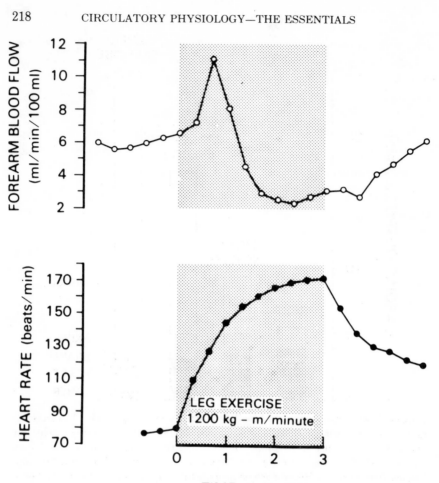

Figure 12-3. Changes in forearm blood flow during severe leg exercise in human subjects. After a temporary increase in forearm (muscle) flow during leg exercise, there was a constriction and flow reduction to about 50% of control. (From B. S. Bevegard and J. T. Shepherd, *J. Appl. Physiol.* 21:123, 1966.)

metabolic activity in the active muscles, the Pco_2, H^+ ion concentration and blood temperature are all considerably increased in the tissues with a resultant shift of the O_2 dissociation curve to the right; this facilitates the release of O_2 to the tissues. The accumulation in muscle of certain metabolites, *e.g.*, K^+, lactic acid and H^+ ions during exhausting exercise is thought to be the main factor responsible for local discomfort, muscle pain and fatigue. The increase in blood lactate reflects the anaerobic breakdown of glucose necessary to maintain the exercise; the capacity to develop an O_2 debt is important in achieving maximal work. Plasma catecholamines increase markedly depending on the intensity of the exercise, a reflection of the sympathetic hyperactivity which is a characteristic of the exercise response.

Physical Training

Repeated physical exercise will induce significant training effects which markedly alter the body's ability to perform work. A minimum regimen necessary to achieve such effects would be two to three exercise sessions per week at 60% $\dot{V}o_{2max}$ for a minimum period of 8 to 10 weeks. Many studies on normal people, trained athletes and animals trained to exercise, have indicated that during such "conditioning," important metabolic and circulatory adaptations are made. The changes are most marked in those individuals who start training at a low fitness level. There is currently widespread interest in physical training effects with particular reference to their possible preventive and therapeutic role in certain cardiovascular disorders, especially ischemic heart disease.

In man, especially in the obese subject, physical training reduces body weight and body fat percentage, increases lean body mass and causes a general reduction in the "fat envelope." Also—very importantly—it will produce a significant improvement in work capacity. This is evidenced by increases in $\dot{V}o_{2max}$ which, in the average individual, can range from 15 to 30%. The rise in $\dot{V}o_2$ is due mainly to the elevation in CO (usually about 20 to 25%) and only to a limited extent to an increase in the A-V O_2 difference.

Trained individuals have better circulatory adaptation to heat, can achieve higher O_2 debts and at the same work level will have lesser accumulation of blood lactate (Fig. 12-4).

From a circulatory standpoint, important changes occur in HR and SV as a result of training. In the normal individual, resting HR is influenced by age, body position (Chapter 13), level of fitness and environmental factors (*e.g.*, altitude and temperature); resting HR becomes progressively less with better physical fitness and will become greater with increasing temperature and altitude. At the same work

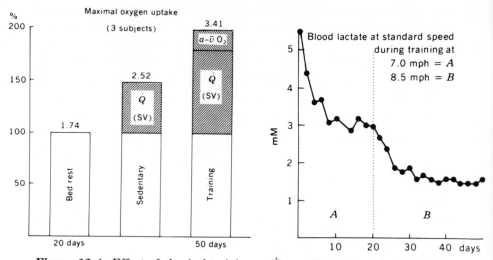

Figure 12-4. Effect of physical training on $\dot{V}O_{2max}$ (L/min) and blood lactate (mM/L) during exercise. *Left,* comparison of $\dot{V}O_{2max}$ of normal subjects after 20 days bed rest, while sedentary and after 50 days of physical training. *Right,* progressive decrease of blood lactate for a standard exercise: *A,* during first 20 days of training, and *B,* during next 30 days of training. (From P. Astrand and K. Rodahl, *Textbook of Work Physiology.* New York: McGraw-Hill Book Co., 1977.)

load, the "conditioned" individual will have a lesser HR and a more rapid postexercise HR recovery; however, his HR_{max} will be unaffected. With training, SV will be increased at rest and at both submaximal and maximal exercise.

There are conflicting reports on the effects of physical training on arterial blood pressure. Endurance athletes usually have a lower systolic pressure at rest and at various levels of exercise. The fit subject often has a lower diastolic pressure during exercise, probably as a manifestation of his greater ability to decrease the peripheral vascular resistance of the arterioles in his exercising muscles. There is some evidence, as yet only fragmentary, that prolonged physical training will reduce arterial blood pressure in hypertensive patients.

Animal studies have indicated that prolonged physical conditioning will result in increased myocardial fiber mass, increased capillary/fiber ratio, improved myocardial contractility and increased coronary artery size. The cardiac hypertrophy of the human endurance athlete also occurs in the physically trained animal, and with it there is improved hemodynamic performance. The evidence on the formation of new collateral vessels in the myocardium is conflicting; however, one definitive study indicates that the effect of ischemia on opening new capillaries is enhanced in the physically-trained heart, suggesting that training plays at least an adjunctive role in promoting new capillary formation. It is, however, very significant that almost all of the above training effects occurred mainly in young animals and only to a very limited extent in older ones, suggesting that physical training, if it is to have lasting effects, might have to be started at an early age.

The mechanisms for the above-described responses to training, particularly the increase in $\dot{V}O_{2max}$, are not certain but are probably due to a combination of an increased oxygen delivery to the muscles (mainly increase in CO) and an increase in the size and number of muscle mitochondria (*i.e.*, increased oxidative capacity of the muscle cell). It is interesting, however, that one training effect, *viz.*, bradycardia, if achieved with repetitive exercise of certain large muscle groups, is operative only when the same trained muscles were used and did not occur with exercise involving the untrained muscles. These findings would suggest that peripheral mechanisms were involved and that cross-adaptation was minimal.

It has been pointed out that physical fitness has important psychological correlates; some studies have shown that physical training can attenuate emotional stress and improve psychological function and social adjustment. However, there is as yet only limited data on this question.

Recent investigations have shown that most patients who have undergone physical training after their myocardial infarct can achieve performance levels at least equivalent to that of normal, sedentary subjects; however, the response to training is often restricted in patients with more extensive infarcts, presumably because of reduced myocardial function. The obvious beneficial effects of supervised physical exercise for coronary patients has prompted increased efforts to provide the much needed physical rehabilitation programs for such patients.

It is now evident that in the case of many coronary patients, their ability to achieve a well-adjusted and productive future life will largely depend on a well-planned and well-executed physical training rehabilitation program.

Exercise Stress Tests

The use of exercise as a screening test in cardiac disease has grown enormously in the last 10 years and has become common procedure in cardiovascular medicine. The primary purposes are (1) to reveal latent ischemic heart disease and (2) to determine the functional capacity of the circulatory system.

While there are numerous test procedures, the most common in the United States is a prescribed treadmill test with progressive levels of physical work, designed to bring the subject to his limit of work capacity. Within narrow limits, each work level requires a specific O_2 uptake per kg body weight per min; thus $\dot{V}_{O_{2max}}$ may be estimated from the stage of the test at which the subject reaches his highest work level (Fig. 12-5). For example, if the subject is forced to stop at the end of the third stage of the Bruce test, *i.e.*, at 3.4 mph at a 14% grade (Fig. 12-5) his $\dot{V}_{O_{2max}}$ will be about 35 ml O_2/kg/min which is about average for middle-aged sedentary American men. Within such a group (of sedentary healthy subjects or functional class I patients), a $\dot{V}_{O_{2max}}$ of 42 ml O_2/kg/min would be an above-average fitness level (Fig. 12-5). As previously mentioned, $\dot{V}_{O_2}$ and heart rate are closely related so that an alternate method to express physical fitness would be the work level at which the subject attains his "target HR."

Each individual has a definable HR_{max}, which declines progressively with age. The average HR_{max}, which is about 190/min at age 20, will decrease to about 165/min at age 60. By setting the mean age-predicted HR_{max} (or 90% of HR_{max}) as a reasonable end-point or "target" HR, it can be determined if the individual can achieve a normal, or near normal, HR_{max}, *i.e.*, has a normal or near normal work capacity.

The presence of cardiac disease is not always easy to distinguish from poor physical condition. Coronary disease is suggested by inability to achieve maximum HR, by abnormal increase in arterial pressure during exercise, by high values of the A-V O_2 difference or by unusually high levels of plasma catecholamines for the exercise level achieved.

However, much more specific evidence for ischemic heart disease is the characteristic anginal pain (described in Chapter 14) or a 1-mm or more displacement of the S-T segment on the exercise ECG. Even

FUNCTIONAL CLASS	CLINICAL STATUS			O₂ REQUIREMENTS ml O_2/kg/min	STEP TEST NAGLE, BALKE, NAUGHTON* 2 min stages 30 steps/min	TREAD-MILL BRUCE[†] 3-min stages	BICYCLE ERGOMETER** For 70 kg body weight kgm/min
NORMAL AND I	PHYSICALLY ACTIVE SUBJECTS			52.5			
				49.0		mph %gr	1500
				45.5	Height (cm)	4.2 16	
				42.0	40		1350
		SEDENTARY HEALTHY		38.5	36		1200
				35.0	32	3.4 14	1050
				31.5	28		
				28.0	24		900
II			DISEASED, RECOVERED	24.5	20	2.5 12	750
			SYMPTOMATIC PATIENTS	21.0	16		600
				17.5	12	1.7 10	450
III				14.0	8		300
				10.5	4		150
				7.0			
IV				3.5			

Figure 12-5. Oxygen requirements (ml/kg/min) at different stages of three standard physical stress tests, *i.e.*, step test, Bruce treadmill test and bicycle ergometer test. The maximum work level achieved defines the $\dot{V}_{O_{2}max}$. The left hand columns show functional classification of normal subjects or patients.

* Nagle, F. S., Balke, B., Naughton, J. P.: Gradational step tests for assessing work capacity. *J. Appl. Physiol.* 20:745–748, 1965.

† Bruce, R. A.: Multi-stage treadmill test of submaximal and maximal exercise. Appendix B, *Exercise Testing and Training of Apparently Healthy Individuals: A Physician's Handbook,* American Heart Association, 1972.

** Fox, S. M., Naughton, J. P., Haskell, W. L.: Physical activity and the prevention of coronary heart disease. *Ann. Clin. Res.* 3:404, 1971.

(Reprinted with permission from *Exercise Testing and Training of Apparently Healthy Individuals: A Handbook for Physicians,* American Heart Association, 1972.)

these signs, while highly suggestive, are not absolute since in both cases false positive or false negatives may occur in 10 to 15% of the cases. As shown in Figure 12-6, S-T displacement of 1 mm or more occurs in a high percentage of patients with angina but also in a significant percentage of the normal population (Fig. 12-6).

One difficulty in the diagnosis of coronary disease (particularly milder disease) is that a degree of coronary sclerosis as well as some decrease in cardiac functional ability is inherent with normal aging. In this regard, Bruce and coworkers have suggested that the response alterations in maximal exercise caused by cardiovascular disease and those attributable to aging can be separated by comparison with age-predicted values for healthy subjects. Deviations from the predicted norm in HR_{max} would suggest deficiencies in $\dot{V}O_{2max}$, *i.e.*, work capacity; deviations in systolic pressure-HR (double) product values would suggest myocardial $\dot{V}O_2$ or left ventricular deficiencies (Chapter 11). Residual differences between these two values would represent peripheral circulatory impairment. These investigators have found this approach useful in separating a deficiency in circulatory delivery of oxygen into left ventricular and peripheral components.

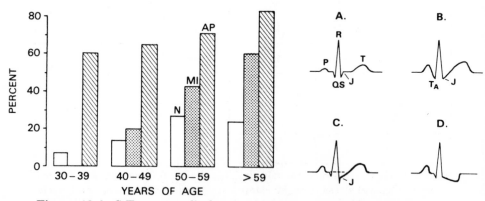

Figure 12-6. S-T segment displacement in myocardial ischemia. *Left*, prevalence of S-T segment depression after maximal exercise in normal subjects, *N*, patients with healed myocardial infarcts, *MI*, and patients with angina pectoris, *AP*. Note the relative independence of age in angina patients but age-dependence in other groups. *Right*, types of S-T changes in exercise: *A*, normal ECG, *B*, false junctional *J* depression due to atrial T wave, *C*, true junctional S-T depression, *D*, S-T downslope segment depression. (From E. Simonson, *Physiology of Work Capacity and Fatigue.* Springfield, Ill.: Charles C Thomas, Publisher, 1971.)

STATIC (ISOMETRIC) EXERCISE

In static (isometric) exercise, the energy expenditure is small compared to dynamic (isotonic) work, but the hemodynamic changes are equally pronounced. Experimentally, static exercise is often induced through maintenance of a sustained handgrip contraction at 30% of maximum voluntary tension to fatigue, which for most subjects is about 4 to 7 minutes. The sustained contraction calls forth a powerful cardiovascular reflex which results in a marked increase in both systolic and diastolic pressure.

If the responses to dynamic and static exercises are contrasted, it will be seen that in both cases there are large increases in systolic pressure; however, in dynamic exercise the increase in HR is much greater and the response of diastolic pressure much less (Fig. 12-7).

In static exercise there is usually an increase in cardiac output, due

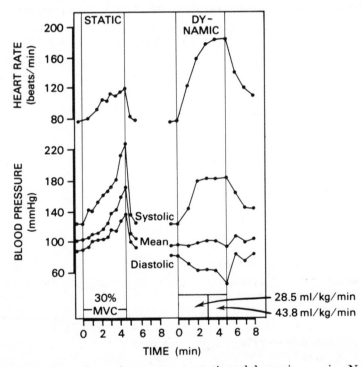

Figure 12-7. Hemodynamic response to static and dynamic exercise. Note in dynamic exercise the much greater rise in heart rate and pulse pressure. (From A. R. Lind and G. W. McNicol, *Canadian Med. Assn. J.* 96: 706, 1967.)

mainly to the heart rate increase; because of the high afterload there is also a sizable increase in stroke work. Plasma catecholamines and blood lactate are elevated.

The blood pressure response is proportional to the intensity of muscle contraction; thus a sustained contraction of 50% of maximal tension will elicit a greater blood pressure response than a 30% maximal contraction (Fig. 12-8). A unique feature of static exercise is that the blood pressure response, while dependent on the intensity and duration of muscle contraction, is independent of the mass of the contracting muscle. Several reports have shown that a sustained contraction of a very small muscle such as the adductor of the little finger will—at the same percentage of maximal tension—elicit the same blood pressure and heart rate response as does a static contraction of the combined musculature of both lower extremities.

It is currently believed that two mechanisms are operative in this powerful CV reflex, *i.e.*, a central cerebral factor and a peripheral reflex

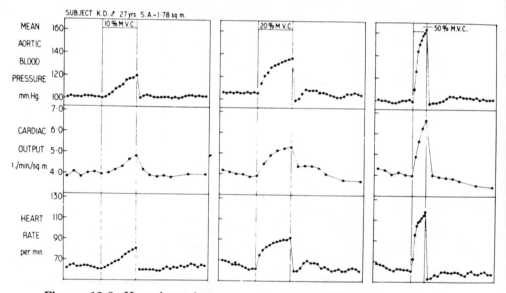

Figure 12-8. Hemodynamic response to sustained handgrip contraction. Mean aortic blood pressure, cardiac output and heart rate before, during and after different degrees of contractile tension, *i.e.*, 10, 20 and 50% of maximum voluntary contraction. The degree of tension is the main factor which significantly influences the hemodynamic response. (From A. R. Lind, S. H. Taylor, P. O. Humphreys, B. M. Kennelly, and K. W. Donald, *Clin. Sci.* 27:229, 1964.)

factor. The cerebral, or "central command" factor is a direct effect of the motor cortex on medullary CV centers, which probably initiate the blood pressure rise; the reflex factor originates in the contracting muscle itself (perhaps due to the liberation of K^+ ions) and apparently assists in increasing the pressure.

At lower muscle tensions (30 to 40% of maximum), the blood flow to the contracting muscles is increased but at higher tensions (70% or more) the blood flow is stopped by the muscle compression. It has been suggested that the blood pressure increase is a compensatory attempt to maintain flow to the ischemic contracting muscle. Lifting and carrying weights can elicit a hemodynamic reflex similar to the standard isometric test; *e.g.*, carrying or holding a 20-kg suitcase for 2½ minutes can induce a systolic blood pressure increase of about 45 mm Hg, a diastolic rise of about 30 mm Hg and a HR increase of about 24/min. There seems little question but that the circulatory response to static exercise, because of its strong diastolic pressure effect, greatly increases cardiac work and contributes importantly to fatigue.

Isometric exercise has been used as a myocardial stress test during cardiac catheterization; patients with cardiac disease but with normal ventricular function at rest, often develop ventricular pressure and wall motion abnormalities during static exercise which help to uncover latent myocardial disease.

EFFECTS OF AGING

Aging and the Cardiovascular System

By 1980 there will be 24 million Americans over 65 years of age—more than 10% of the population. In this group, cardiovascular disease is the most frequent cause of hospitalization and death. Not only does the incidence of cardiovascular disease increase steeply with age but there is (as mentioned previously) a striking similarity between the effects of age *per se* and early coronary heart disease. This sometimes poses a serious problem in differential diagnosis and makes it particularly important to establish norms for cardiovascular function in the aged before reaching conclusions regarding cardiovascular pathology.

At rest there are only minor changes in cardiac function with age. However, with exercise, older individuals show significant differences in their circulatory responsiveness. In adults, $\dot{V}O_{2max}$ tends to be highest at about age 27 and, thereafter, steadily decreases so that at age 65 it is about 60% of the former value (Fig. 12-9).

It has been reported that the rate of decrease of $\dot{V}O_{2max}$ is three times greater in the sedentary individual and also more rapid in the obese and the smoker. This limitation in work capacity is not in the respiratory or neuromuscular system nor in arterial oxygen content or A-V O_2 extraction, but lies in the ability to transport O_2, *i.e.*, in the circulation.

Hemodynamic Changes with Age

Older men and women respond to exercise with progressively lesser increases in HR, SV and CO and greater increases in systolic pressure. With exercise, it is also significant that the elderly have elevated pulmonary arterial wedge pressures and increased right ventricular end-diastolic pressures, suggesting a diminished reserve capacity in older hearts.

Age changes have also been studied in different animal species using

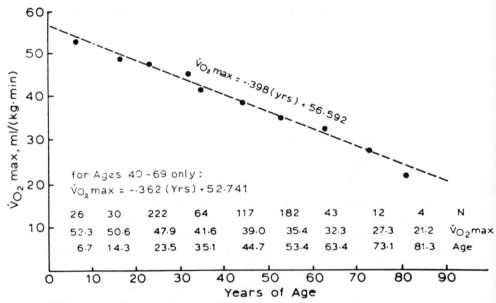

Figure 12-9. Regression of mean $\dot{V}O_{2max}$ per decade of age in 700 boys and men, corrected for body weight showing a steady decline of oxygen uptake during maximal exercise with advancing age. (From M. M. Dehn and R. A. Bruce, *J. Appl. Physiol.* 33:805, 1972.)

both isolated organs and organs *in situ*; this permits analysis of systems free of peripheral vascular and neurohumoral influences. Such studies have revealed that the aged myocardium can develop comparable degrees of active tension and peak tension but takes a longer time to develop the tensions; there is, therefore, an increased duration of both contraction and relaxation periods. These contractile deficits are thought to be due in part to a greater stiffness of the myocardial wall because of viscoelastic changes in the muscle fibers and in part to the lesser ability of the muscle to respond adequately to catecholamines during stress (Fig. 12-10).

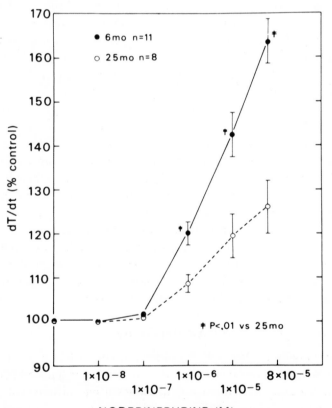

NOREPINEPHRINE (M)

Figure 12-10. The effect of age on the maximal rate of myocardial tension development (dT/dt) to increasing concentration of norepinephrine in old and young rats. (From E. G. Lakatta, G. Gerstenblith, C. S. Angell, N. W. Shock, and M. L. Weisfelt, *Circ. Res.* 36:262, 1975. By permission of the American Heart Association.)

Interestingly enough, there are apparently no differences in myocardial length-tension curves with age so that the heterometric response seems relatively unaffected; however, the lesser response to norepinephrine would seem to be an important handicap. There is also increasing stiffness of heart valves and pericardium, which may have important consequences for cardiac function.

It has been consistently observed that in man, peripheral resistance at rest and at comparable work loads is increased with age and that in exercise there is a lesser dilator capability of vascular smooth muscle.

It is well known that in both older animals and man, there is a decreased arterial distensibility, *i.e.*, increasing stiffness of the aorta and large arteries in both a radial and longitudinal direction as determined by pressure-volume curves (Chapter 1). Accompanying this, especially after age 60, is an increase in aortic volume which preserves, to some extent, the hemodynamic buffering capacity of the aorta and minimizes the pressure changes due to ventricular ejection. With increasing age, there is a progressive rise in arterial pressure (Chapter 4) and evidence of decreased venous compliance.

The increased stiffness of the large arteries and the loss of the diastolic rebound serve to increase the mechanical impedance of the aortic bed; these changes along with the increased peripheral vascular resistance impose a heavier afterload on the heart. The increased impedance to ejection may be the factor limiting the increase in stroke volume in the aging ventricle. It should be noted that the arterial rigidity is mainly a result of a diffuse process involving the replacement of elastin with connective tissue; the result is due to an alteration of viscoelastic properties of the wall at large and not to atherosclerosis, which is generally a patchy and irregular process.

Autonomic Responsiveness and Aging

As previously mentioned, the older individual has a distinctly impaired response to physical exercise both from a cardiac and peripheral vascular standpoint. While there are associated pathological changes in the cardiovascular tissues, it is not certain to what extent the functional deficiencies in the intact, older individual are due to local changes in tissue performance, to defective autonomic reflexes or to insufficient neurohumoral stimulation during stress.

Autonomic stress tests in normal subjects of different ages have shown a lesser rise in heart rate and in diastolic pressure in the older subjects during head-up tilt, and lesser heart rate increments to the standard Valsalva test. Whether the defect lies in the afferent or efferent limb of the autonomic reflex is not known. Studies in animals and man indicate that the baroceptors may become less sensitive with advancing age (Fig. 12-11).

It has been suggested that this decreased baroceptor sensitivity may be due to increased rigidity of the aorta and carotid arteries which would result in lesser deformation of the receptors and less stimulation for equivalent pressure changes. Tissue studies have also indicated that aged myocardium has a decreased catecholamine content and also a lesser inotropic responsiveness to catecholamines (Fig. 12-10);

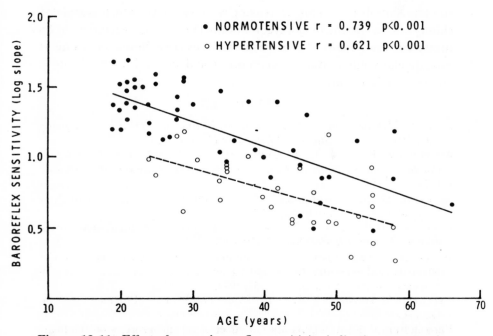

Figure 12-11. Effect of age on baroreflex sensitivity indicating a progressive fall in the sensitivity index (pulse interval/Δ systolic pressure) with increasing age in both normotensives and hypertensives. (From B. Gribbin, T. G. Pickering, P. Sleight, and R. Peto, *Circ. Res.* 39:424, 1971. By permission of the American Heart Association.)

the latter action is apparently due to impaired ability of catecholamines to adequately increase the calcium supply of contracting muscle.

With regard to general sympathoadrenal response, recent studies in man have shown that norepinephrine levels increase with age and that older subjects have a greater increase in norepinephrine in response to standard stresses such as exercise and upright posture.

In summary, it might be said that studies thus far, admittedly rather limited, seem to indicate that with advancing age: (a) there are pathological anatomic changes in the aorta and large arteries which result in heightened vascular impedance and increased work loads on the heart; (b) the myocardium becomes less distensible and has longer contraction and relaxation periods. Functionally, these changes are associated with (c) a steadily decreasing work capacity, the rate of decrease being heavily dependent on individual factors such as physical training and obesity. This decreasing work capacity, which correlates closely with a diminishing oxygen uptake ($\dot{V}o_{2max}$), is accompanied by primary hemodynamic defects, especially decrease in maximum heart rate, stroke volume and cardiac output and increasing end-diastolic and arterial blood pressures.

REFERENCES

AMERICAN HEART ASSOCIATION: *Exercise Testing and Training of Apparently Healthy Individuals: A Physicians Handbook*, 1972.

AMSTERDAM, E. A., J. H. WILMORE, AND A. N. DeMARIA: *Exercise in Cardiovascular Health and Disease*. New York: Yorke Medical Books, 1977.

ASTRAND, P., AND K. RODAHL: *Textbook of Work Physiology*, 2nd ed. New York: McGraw-Hill Book Co., 1977.

BEVEGARD, B. S., AND J. T. SHEPHERD: Regulation of circulation during exercise in man. *Physiol. Rev.* 47:178, 1967.

BRUCE, R. A., L. D. FISHER, M. N. COOPER, AND G. O. GEY: Separation of effects of cardiovascular disease and age on ventricular function with maximal exercise. *Am. J. Cardiol.* 34:757, 1974.

ELLESTAD, M. H.: *Stress Testing: Principles and Practice*. Philadelphia: F. A. Davis Co., 1976.

FROELICHER, V. F.: Animal studies of effect of chronic exercise on the heart and atherosclerosis: A review. *Am. Heart J.* 84:496, 1972.

GERSTENBLITH, G., E. G. LAKATTA, AND M. L. WEISFELDT: Age changes in myocardial function and exercise response. *Prog. Cardiovasc. Dis.* 19:1, 1976.

JUDY, W. V.: Physiology of Exercise. In *Physiology,* ed. by E. E. Selkurt. Boston: Little, Brown and Co., 1976.

KALBFLEISCH, J. H., J. A. REINKE, C. J. PORTH, T. J. EBERT, AND J. J. SMITH: Effect of age on circulatory response to postural and Valsalva tests. *Proc. Soc. Exp. Biol. Med.* 156:100, 1977.

LIND, A. R., AND G. W. MCNICOL. Circulatory responses to sustained handgrip contractions performed during other exercise both rhythmic and static. *J. Physiol.* 192:575, 1967.

MARSHALL, R. J., AND J. T. SHEPHERD: *Cardiac Function in Health and Disease.* Philadelphia: W. B. Saunders Co., 1968.

MCDERMOTT, D. J., W. J. STEKIEL, J. J. BARBORIAK, L. C. KLOTH AND J. J. SMITH. The effect of age on hemodynamic and metabolic response to static exercise. *J. Appl. Physiol.* 37:923, 1974.

MITCHELL, J. H., AND K. WILDENTHAL: Static isometric exercise and the heart. *Annu. Rev. Med.* 25:369, 1974.

SCHEUER, J., AND C. M. TIPTON: Cardiovascular adaptations to physical training. *Annu. Rev. Physiol.* 39:221, 1977.

SIMONSON, E.: *Physiology of Work Capacity and Fatigue.* Springfield, Ill.: Charles C Thomas, Publisher, 1971.

STRANDELL, T.: Circulatory studies on healthy old men. *Acta Med. Scand.* 175:Suppl. 414, 1964.

VATNER, S. F., AND M. PAGANI: Cardiovascular adjustments to exercise. *Prog. Cardiovasc. Dis.* 19:91, 1976.

chapter 13

Circulatory Response to Non-exercise Stress

Stress is the result of a real or imagined threat to the well-being of the individual; it usually involves the autonomic nervous system and if sufficiently serious, there is activation of the defense center of the hypothalamus with a powerful sympathoadrenal release (Chapter 10). Individuals vary widely in their responses to stress depending upon their age, physical and emotional state and the nature and severity of the stress. The effects of physical exercise, both dynamic and static, as well as the principles of exercise stress testing were discussed in Chapter 12.

In this chapter are included brief descriptions of a few common non-exercise physical stresses and the clinical tests which are sometimes used to simulate them. Because inadequate reactions to such tests are often the first signs of impending disease, compensatory stress responses and their mechanisms will be analyzed.

POSTURAL AND GRAVITY EFFECTS ON THE CIRCULATION

Normal Postural Responses

For normal man, standing erect presents no problem but an inadequate orthostatic response may be an indication of a serious clinical disturbance. The upright posture requires proper functioning and coordination of the musculoskeletal system, the nervous system and the circulatory system. From a circulatory standpoint the two main elements concerned in postural abnormalities are the skeletal muscle pump and the baroceptor reflexes.

Postural changes are often simulated through use of a tilt table or by "lower body negative pressure," a procedure in which air is evacuated and pressure reduced in a box enclosing the lower body below the iliac crests. These devices produce hemodynamic changes virtually identical to standing erect and have the advantage of facilitating physiological measurements. Such investigations have shown that with 70° head-up tilt, there is in a normal adult, a rapid, caudal shift of about 500 to 700 ml of thoracic venous blood; this results in a decrease in venous return (of about 20%), stroke volume (about 40%) and cardiac output (about 15 to 20%). The amount of translocated central venous blood is, therefore, roughly equivalent to that removed in a standard phlebotomy (500 ml of blood withdrawal from a peripheral vein). A typical response pattern is shown in Figure 13-1.

As the central blood volume and cardiac output decrease and the arterial pressure begins to fall, there is a strong vasoconstriction, particularly of the splanchnic, renal and skeletal muscle beds, with a consequent net rise in total peripheral resistance. The increases in resistance (about 40%) and in heart rate (about 20%) not only maintain but increase the diastolic and mean arterial pressure (about 10%). Systolic pressure shows little or no change.

These cardiac and resistance changes are reflex responses of the arterial and cardiopulmonary baroceptors; curiously enough, venoconstriction is transient and limited. Within a few minutes of standing, the plasma norepinephrine and epinephrine concentrations are elevated about 4-fold from their control levels of about 165 and 16 pg/ml of plasma respectively. The plasma vasopressin concentration is increased about 10 to 15% upon standing.

Although the blood pressure and heart rate changes are fairly

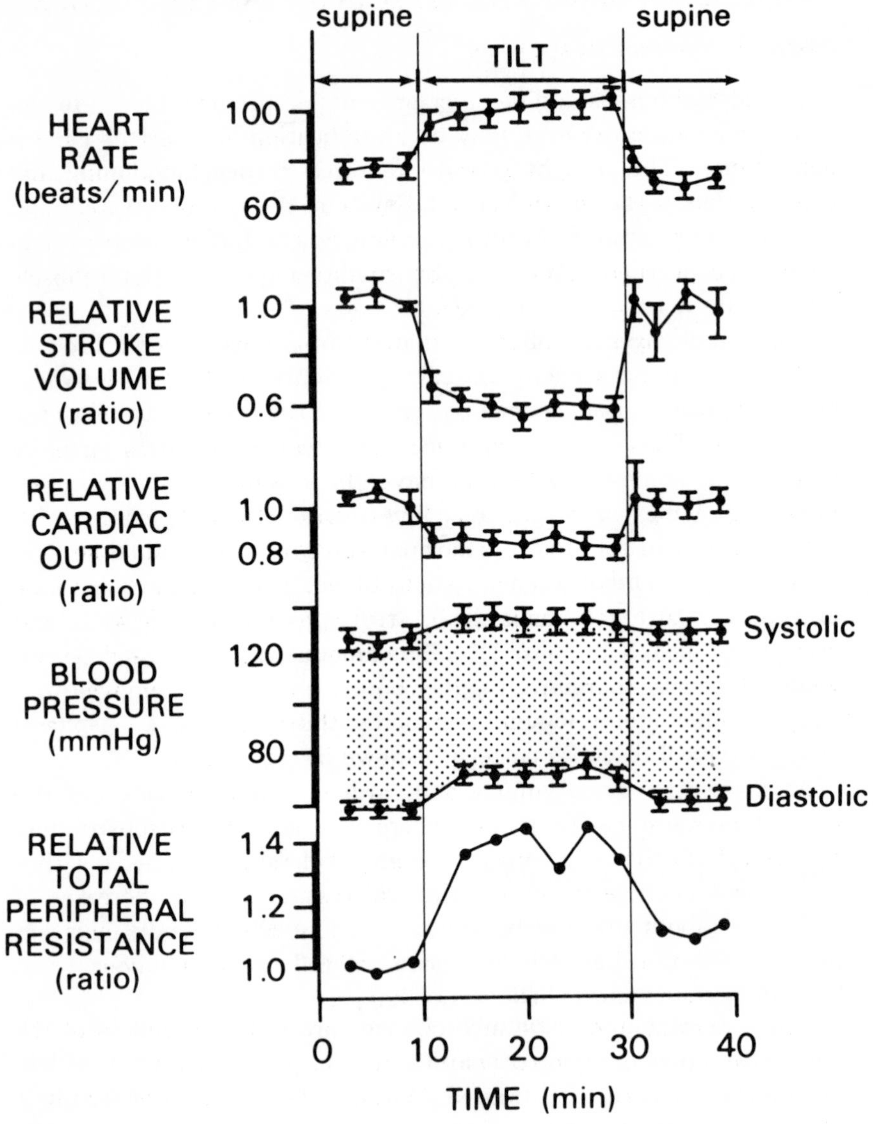

Figure 13-1. Response of normal young men to a 20-minute head-up tilt showing means and standard error of means. Note the prompt increase in heart rate, vascular resistance and diastolic pressure and the decrease in stroke volume, cardiac output and pulse pressure. (From J. J. Smith, J. E. Bush, V. T. Wiedmeier, and F. E. Tristani, *J. Appl. Physiol.* 29:133, 1970.)

consistent among normal individuals of similar age, other parameters show variations; *e.g.*, in some cases blood pressure is maintained with only a small decrease in cardiac output and a modest increase in peripheral resistance; however, in other subjects there is a greater fall in stroke volume and cardiac output and a larger rise in peripheral resistance. The significance of such variations is not known at present. With advancing age there is a tendency toward lesser increases in heart rate and diastolic pressure during head-up tilt (Chapter 12).

With prolonged standing, the renal vasoconstriction leads to a progressive decrease in renal blood flow and consequently a sharp increase in plasma renin, angiotensin and plasma aldosterone levels—hormonal changes which help to maintain plasma volume. In the upright position there is a 20% decrease in cerebral blood flow and, for reasons which are not clear, a hyperventilation, with a tendency toward hypocapnea; this combination of factors undoubtedly contributes to the 5 to 10% fainting rate usually encountered during prolonged postural tests.

As stated in Chapter 4, the upright posture will not alter the pressure gradient between the arterial and venous beds but will increase the transmural pressure in vessels below the heart; *e.g.*, pressure in the foot veins will rise by 80 to 90 mm Hg when standing. As a result there may be an increased transfer of fluid into the interstitial space producing a mild edema of the feet, even in normal individuals, after several hours of standing; heat exaggerates this effect.

Abnormal Postural Responses

Decreased tolerance to the upright posture will occur if the skeletal muscle pump effect on venous return is inadequate (Chapter 4) or if the baroceptor reflexes (Chapter 10) are interrupted. The latter may occur (a) in certain systemic diseases such as diabetes or syphilis, (b) in primary idiopathic hypotension, or (c) after administration of adrenergic blocking agents. Such patients, upon standing or being tilted, experience a rapid fall in blood pressure and often faint abruptly without the usual premonitory symptoms of pallor, sweating and nausea.

Transient postural hypotension will also occur after prolonged bed rest, water immersion of 6 hours or longer or exposure to the weightless or zero gravity state (Fig. 13-2). The hypotension in these situations has been attributed to the decreased plasma volume (common in these conditions) and to the lessened gravity effect on the arterial baroceptors. The latter explanation seems less likely since gravity changes affect all parts of the body equally, and theoretically should not influence the arterial stretch induced by internal pressure changes.

Cardiac patients with congestive failure may show increased tolerance to postural stress, and head-up tilt may result in an increased stroke volume and cardiac output associated with relief of dyspnea (Fig. 13-3). It has been suggested that this paradoxical effect may be associated with a leftward shift of the failing heart on the "Starling curve" to relative compensation, permitting an increased stroke volume at lesser filling pressures.

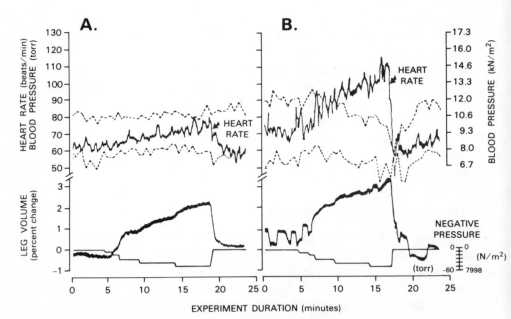

Figure 13-2. Response of skylab commander to lower body negative pressure test before (A) and on 20th day (B) of zero gravity. In B there is a greater rise in heart rate and decrease in blood pressure during LBNP; with the sudden fall in heart rate, fainting was imminent and the test was discontinued. (From R. L. Johnson, G. W. Hoffler, A. E. Nicogossian, S. A. Bergman, and M. M. Jackson, *Third Manned Skylab Mission*, NASA Tech Memo TMX 58154, Nov., 1974.)

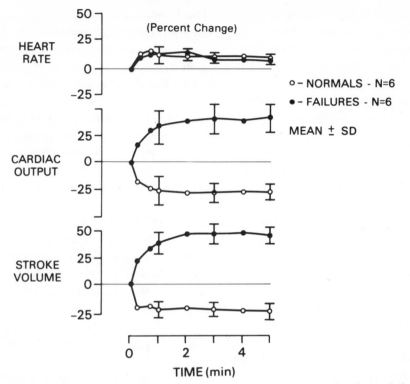

Figure 13-3. Comparison of hemodynamic response of congestive heart failure patients and normal subjects to head-up tilt. In contrast to the normal subjects, note the increased stroke volume and cardiac output in the patients. (Courtesy Dr. W. V. Judy, University of Indiana, unpublished data.)

Recent reports have also indicated that some borderline hypertensive patients have increased cardiac output and exaggerated diastolic pressure responses to head-up tilt (Chapter 15).

INCREASED INTRATHORACIC PRESSURE (THE VALSALVA TEST)

Normal Valsalva Responses

In 1707 the Italian anatomist, Valsalva, described a maneuver in which the subject closes the mouth and nose, expires forcibly and thereby increases the pressure inside the pharynx and lung passages. The original purpose was to inflate the middle ear *via* the eustachian tubes; today the test is more commonly used as a means of assessing autonomic responsiveness to circulatory changes. By increasing intrathoracic pressure and thereby impeding venous return, cardiac output and arterial pressure are reduced; the resulting hemodynamic strain tests the circulatory system and particularly the integrity of the autonomic circulatory reflexes.

As commonly carried out, the subject expires against a 40 mm Hg resistance for 15 seconds; there is a sudden rise in intrathoracic, intraabdominal and cerebrospinal fluid pressure. The peripheral venous valves shut, and the blood, prevented from flowing into the vena cavae, accumulates in the peripheral veins. Aortic flow drops to about 50% of control.

The Valsalva response is classically divided into four phases as illustrated in Figure 13-4. At the start of the strain (phase I) there is a sudden rise in arterial pressure as the heightened intrathoracic pressure is transmitted directly through the aorta to the arterial tree; the heart rate usually shows a small decrease. In phase II there is diminished venous return to the right heart; cardiac filling becomes inadequate and the mean arterial and pulse pressures begin to fall; then follow a reflex tachycardia and peripheral vasoconstriction which limit the pressure drop. In phase III, immediately after release, blood pressure drops quickly because of the sudden fall in intrathoracic pressure and the heart rate increases further. In phase IV the blood pressure rebounds as a result of the rapid surge of venous return, and in about 5 to 6 seconds overshoots, reflexly inducing a marked bradycardia (Fig. 13-4).

The Valsalva test simulates the type of stress often associated with lifting, pushing, blowing a musical instrument, straining at stool, coughing *etc.* The maneuver tests the ability of the circulatory system to cope with a decreasing venous return and a falling arterial pressure and thus is a measure of the integrity of the baroceptor and cardiopulmonary reflexes.

Abnormal Valsalva Responses

Most clinical abnormalities of the Valsalva are due either to (a) an increased intrathoracic blood volume, or (b) interruption of the baroceptor reflex arc, or (c) a combination of these two.

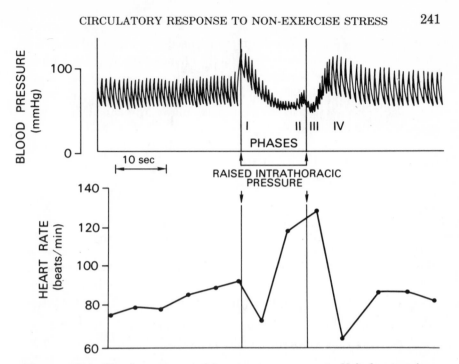

Figure 13-4. Blood pressure and heart rate response to Valsalva test in a normal young adult. Intrathoracic pressure, 40 mm Hg. Note (*upper*) the falling arterial pressure and tachycardia in phase II. The highest (phases II and III) and lowest (phases I and IV) heart rates for the respective phases are shown in the lower figure. The pressure overshoot and bradycardia in phase IV (*upper*) and the large heart rate decrement from phases III to IV (*lower*) indicate functional baroceptor reflexes.

Increase in intrathoracic blood volume occurs in congestive heart failure and results in a "square wave" Valsalva response in which there is little or no change in pulse pressure in phases II and III and very little or no overshoot in phase IV (Fig. 13-5).

The arterial pressure is maintained because (a) the increased central blood volume and atrial filling pressure provide a reservoir of venous return which maintains the cardiac output, and (b) the heightened peripheral venous pressure which usually accompanies the increased central blood volume, reduces venous distensibility and helps maintain a higher venous pressure gradient toward the right atrium. As the congestion lessens, the Valsalva response becomes more normal because of the abatement of these factors.

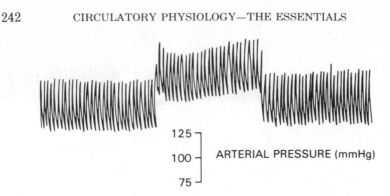

125 ⌉
100 ⌐ ARTERIAL PRESSURE (mmHg)
75 ⌋

Figure 13-5. "Square wave" blood pressure response to the Valsalva test in hypertensive heart failure. There is no change in pulse pressure, no pressure overshoot and very little change in heart rate. (From E. P. Sharpey-Schafer, in *Handbook of Physiology*, Section 2: *Circulation*, vol. III, ed. by W. F. Hamilton and P. Dow. Washington, D.C.: American Physiological Society, 1965.)

Since heart rate, a non-invasive measurement, is reportedly as valid an autonomic indicator as blood pressure, it may also be used to assess the Valsalva response; in the normal individual, the heart rate changes, as might be predicted, are roughly opposite to those of the blood pressure as shown in Figure 13-4. Because in congestive failure, the blood pressure changes are greatly diminished, the heart rate response is also flatter than normal (Fig. 13-6*A*).

Recent reports have indicated that ambulatory coronary heart disease patients not in congestive failure also have decreased heart rate responses to the Valsalva test (Fig. 13-6*B*); this lessened heart rate response may be due either to a subclinical intrathoracic congestion or decreased baroreflex responsiveness.

Interruption of the baroreflex arc may occur in neurological disorders involving the autonomic nervous system such as primary idiopathic hypotension; in such cases, the Valsalva test will show a continued pressure fall in phase II because of the failure of vasoconstriction and cardioacceleration and a lack of arterial pressure rebound and a bradycardia in phase IV (Fig. 13-7); these individuals, as previously mentioned, are also prone to postural hypotension.

DIVING (FACE IMMERSION) REFLEX

This unique reflex represents the ultimate defense of the submerged vertebrate against asphyxia, *i.e.*, a gross redistribution of the circula-

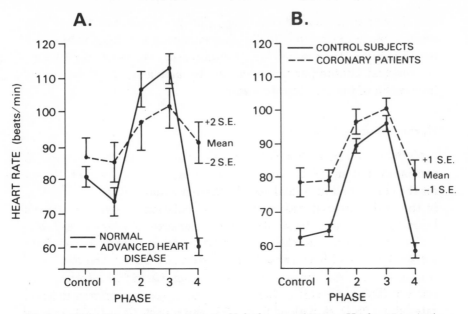

Figure 13-6. Heart rate response to Valsalva test (40 mm Hg for 15 sec): *A*, in congestive heart failure patients (From E. I. Elisberg, *J.A.M.A.* 186:200, 1963); and *B*, coronary patients not in congestive failure. Note in both cases the "flattened" response compared to control subjects. (From F. E. Tristani, D. G. Kamper, D. J. McDermott, B. J. Peters, and J. J. Smith, *Am. J. Physiol.* 233:H694, 1977.)

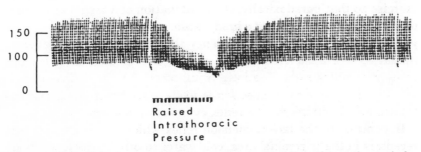

Figure 13-7. Valsalva response in a patient with idiopathic orthostatic hypotension. There is an excessive fall in blood pressure in phase II and an absence of overshoot and bradycardia in phase IV. (From R. H. Johnson and J. M. K. Spalding, *Disorders of the Autonomic Nervous System.* London: Blackwell Scientific Publications, 1974.)

tion in order to concentrate oxygen in the brain and heart. This remarkable response enables the domestic duck to remain submerged for 15 minutes, the sea lion for 30 minutes and the whale for 2 hours. Its residual counterpart in man can be activated by diving or by immersion of the face in cold water.

Hemodynamic Changes

In the duck, hemodynamic changes involve a sudden decrease in cardiac output and heart rate to about 6% of the control values. Except for the coronary and cranial vessels, there is a massive vasoconstriction of the entire arterial tree so that the circulation becomes in effect a heart-brain circuit. The stroke volume and arterial pressure are relatively unchanged; when the animal surfaces, these changes are reversed within seconds with a large overshoot in cardiac output and heart rate (Fig. 13-8). The face immersion reflex in man will induce a comparable but less intense response characterized by a quick reduction in heart rate (about 25%), skin blood flow (75%) and muscle flow (50%). Arterial blood pressure increases by about 20% (Fig. 13-8B).

The key responses are a powerful, all-embracing, peripheral vasoconstriction and an intense vagal bradycardia. Breathholding alone will cause similar, but much less marked effects. The bradycardic effect is greater with cold (rather than cool) water and an attenuated response can be elicited by dry cold. An unusual feature is that the bradycardic effect of face immersion is increased during physical exercise so that paradoxically, the combination of a tachycardic stimulus (dynamic exercise) and a bradycardic stimulus (diving reflex) may yield a stronger bradycardic tendency than diving alone. A response similar to face immersion may be produced by inhalation of noxious gases or smelling salts. The integrating center for the diving reflex is not known; a cerebral connection is likely since threatening motions toward a seal will induce the reflex even before immersion.

In contrast to the face immersion reflex which is activated by cold receptors in the trigeminal area, cold water to other parts of the body causes reflex increases in heart rate and blood pressure; the cold pressor test (Chapter 10), involving immersion of the hand in ice water (0°C), will stimulate pain fibers as well as cold receptors and produce a greater rise in blood pressure and heart rate than cold water (10°C).

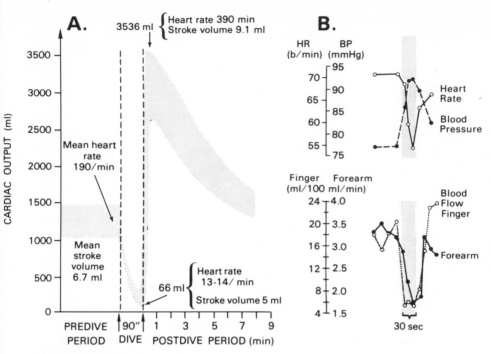

Figure 13-8. Diving and face immersion reflex: *A*, hemodynamic responses to 90-second head submersion in a duck (From B. Folkow, N. J. Nilsson, and L. R. Younce, *Acta Physiol. Scand.* 70:347, 1967); *B*, responses to 30-second face immersion in normal male subjects. (From D. D. Heistad, F. M. Abboud, and J. W. Eckstein, *J. Appl. Physiol.* 25:542, 1968.) In man the decrease in heart rate and blood flow are of lesser degree.

Clinical Implications

Because of the powerful vagal action, pathological arrhythmias such as ventricular premature contraction and idioventricular rhythm, as well as T wave inversions commonly occur after only 30 seconds of diving in man. Because of its vagal effect, this reflex has been used successfully to abort attacks of paroxysmal tachycardia. The face immersion reflex is used as a relatively "pure" test for vagal bradycardia; while sympathetic vasoconstriction is simultaneously activated, the bradycardic effect is relatively immune to other reflex restraints, *e.g.*, by baroceptors or physical exercise. The bradycardic response decreases linearly with age and reportedly is diminished in coronary patients after myocardial infarction, while sympathetic pressor responses remain intact.

HEMORRHAGE

Circulatory Changes in Hemorrhage

The clinical results of blood loss depend on many factors, but particularly on the rate and degree of bleeding, the age and health of the patient and availability of treatment. The blood pressure and general response in an uncomplicated, untreated hemorrhage in a normal adult occurring within a relatively brief period (15 to 30 min) might be roughly estimated as shown in Table 13-1.

The brief description in this section refers mainly to short-term responses to moderate bleeding (less than 30% of blood volume); protracted hemorrhagic hypotension generally leads to circulatory shock, a quite different pathophysiological entity, which will be discussed in Chapter 15.

The immediate consequences of hemorrhage are (a) a decrease in blood volume, (b) a fall in venous return and cardiac output, and (c) a resultant decline in arterial and venous pressure.

Compensatory Response to Hemorrhage

Within seconds after bleeding begins, the fall in central blood volume and arterial pressure will activate cardiopulmonary and baroceptor reflexes (particularly from the carotid sinuses) and as a result, the sympathoadrenal defense system is fully mobilized. In case of a rela-

Table 13-1. Arterial Blood Pressure and Clinical Result of Hemorrhage

Loss of Blood Volume	Mean Arterial Pressure— Immediate Response	Likely Result
10%	Little change	Spontaneous recovery
15 to 20%	80 to 90 mm Hg	Moderate hypotension, spontaneous recovery
20 to 30%	60 to 80 mm Hg	Early shock—usually reversible
30 to 40%	50 to 70 mm Hg	Serious shock— irreversible in some cases

tively small hemorrhage, *e.g.*, a standard phlebotomy of 500 ml, there is a modest rise in peripheral resistance and a small decrease in pulse pressure (Fig. 13-9).

With a greater blood loss and more marked hypotension, the responses will be correspondingly greater. The main compensatory changes are:

1. Increase in Heart Rate and Contractility. Tachycardia does not usually occur, however, in uncomplicated hemorrhage until the blood loss exceeds 700 to 800 ml.

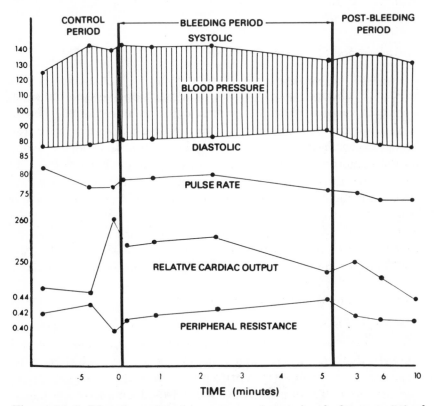

Figure 13-9. Mean hemodynamic response of normal male donors to 540 ml phlebotomy (n = 25). Uncomplicated hemorrhage of about 10% of blood volume. Note the preliminary fall in peripheral resistance and rise in cardiac output just after insertion of the needle and before bleeding was begun. Note also the immediate widening of the pulse pressure as the bleeding is stopped. (From J. R. Logic, S. A. Johnson, and J. J. Smith, *Transfusion* 3:83, 1963.)

2. Strong Generalized Constriction of Both Resistance and Capacitance Vessels. In particular, vessels of skin (producing a marked pallor), splanchnic area (with resulting ischemia of gut and liver), skeletal muscle and kidney are affected. Cerebral and coronary beds are unaffected.

The renal vasoconstriction reduces glomerular filtration leading to oliguria and sometimes to anuria. Venoconstriction is a prominent aspect of the compensatory reaction; in the splanchnic bed for example, which contains about 20% of the total blood volume, a translocation of even half of this amount to the central veins can provide a significant autotransfusion.

Maintenance of Plasma Volume

Vasoconstriction assists the circulation in two ways: (a) by decreasing the circulatory capacity so the remaining blood volume will create a greater venous filling pressure; and (b) by lowering the general capillary hydrostatic pressure and thus promoting fluid transfer from tissues to the plasma. Certain hormonal mechanisms are also activated during hemorrhage to help maintain the plasma volume (Fig. 13-10). Renal vasoconstriction reduces glomerular filtration and urine formation; renin and angiotensin production is increased *via* renal ischemia. The decreased atrial stretch causes reflex release of vasopressin (ADH) and (along with other factors) is responsible for the release of aldosterone from the adrenal cortex. These two hormones maximize H_2O and Na^+ reabsorption from renal tubules and help conserve plasma volume.

Other Responses to Hemorrhage

There is a pronounced increase in plasma catecholamines; epinephrine is responsible for the hyperglycemia in hemorrhage but it is unlikely that any of the circulatory hormones, *i.e.*, catecholamines, angiotensin or vasopressin contribute significantly to the general vasoconstriction. There is a decrease in RBCs, hematocrit and plasma protein concentration in blood because of the dilution by the absorbed tissue fluid. After the hemorrhage, the plasma proteins are usually replaced in about 3 to 6 days and the RBCs in about 4 to 6 weeks. Therapy is logically directed at fluid replacement, whole blood if the hematocrit is low but if not available, plasma or plasma substitutes.

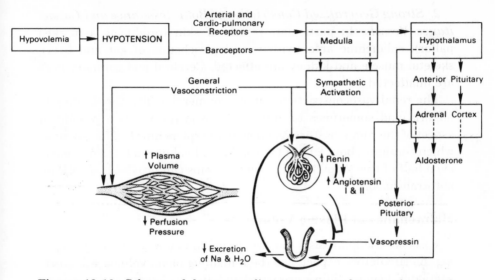

Figure 13-10. Schema of factors tending to restore plasma volume and extracellular fluid during and after hemorrhage. Reduced general capillary pressure and renal vasoconstriction are key elements in maintaining plasma volume; increased vasopressin and aldosterone levels are helpful adjuncts.

FAINTING (SYNCOPE)

Fainting is the <u>loss of consciousness due to cerebral ischemia;</u> clinically a differentiation is usually made between "organic" and "functional" causes. Organic factors would include inadequate baroceptor response due to disease or alpha adrenergic blockade, the latter occurring, *e.g.*, as a side effect of antihypertensive therapy. As previously mentioned, these patients usually faint abruptly upon standing without showing the usual preliminary symptoms.

Functional syncope or ordinary fainting (also called vasodepressor or vasovagal syncope) has multiple causes. It may occur in unusually sensitive individuals after a purely psychic stimulation such as emotional shock or the sight of blood; on the other hand practically everyone will faint during extreme somatic stress such as a 1500-ml phlebotomy or a 60-minute passive, suspended tilt. However, clinical fainting in the healthy individual is usually due to a combination of stresses; the most common predisposing factor is decreased circulating blood volume induced, *e.g.*, by a previous blood withdrawal, excessive physical exercise, diarrhea, protracted bed rest or prolonged standing in the heat.

Circulatory Responses during Fainting

The usual preliminary symptoms of extreme pallor, nausea, sweating and abdominal discomfort are sometimes stated as being due to sympathoadrenal activation but are more likely due to the liberation of vasopressin. These symptoms are usually accompanied by a decreasing systolic and pulse pressure, a rapid heart rate and decreasing right atrial pressure. At the moment of vascular failure, there is a sudden sharp decrease in mean arterial and pulse pressure, a marked bradycardia, cerebral ischemia and loss of consciousness—all occurring very rapidly, sometimes within seconds (Fig. 13-11).

The right atrial pressure usually falls further but cardiac output remains relatively unchanged. The key defect is a powerful vagal stimulation accompanied by a sudden loss of peripheral vascular resistance, primarily in skeletal muscle; the mechanism is probably a massive sympathetic inhibition from the hypothalamic cardioinhibitory center (Chapter 10). Cholinergic vasodilators do not seem to be involved.

Mechanism of Vasodepressor Syncope

While it is generally agreed that the immediate prelude to fainting is cerebral ischemia, there are little data and no unanimity of opinion regarding the final common pathway through which the circulatory collapse is brought about. Because of the unusual autoregulatory ability of cerebral vessels, signs of cerebral ischemia usually do not occur until arterial pressures reach very low levels, i.e., about 40 mm Hg. However, a heightened cerebral arterial tone decreases autoregulatory ability so that cerebral ischemia develops at higher arterial pressures than is usually the case. Two conditions which increase cerebral vascular tone are hypocapnea and hypertension.

Hyperventilation and its resultant hypocapnea commonly occur not only in emotional strain but during hemorrhage and postural stress; the hypocapnea will, in turn, induce tachycardia and increased cardiac output. However, the most striking effect of hypocapnea is the cerebral vasoconstriction which can reduce cerebral flow by 40% after only 1 or

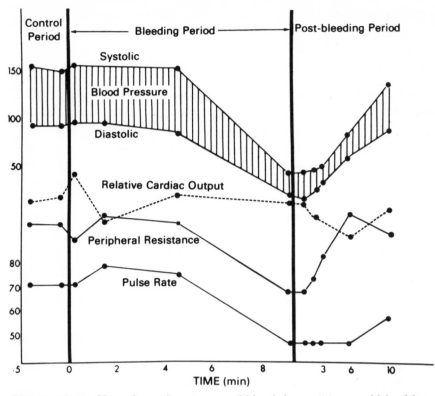

Figure 13-11. Hemodynamic response of blood donor (53-year-old healthy male) to a 580-ml phlebotomy. Toward the end of the bleeding, subject developed pallor, nausea and abdominal discomfort. Blood pressure just before end of bleeding was 46/25. Note the sharp fall in mean and pulse pressure, peripheral resistance and heart rate. Cardiac output was maintained. (From J. R. Logic, S. A. Johnson, and J. J. Smith, *Transfusion* 3:83, 1963.)

2 minutes of active hyperventilation. Although uncomplicated hyperventilation rarely causes syncope in normal subjects, it can be an important contributing factor. Similarly, certain hypertensive patients develop cerebral ischemia at higher than normal levels of arterial pressure and have fainting tendencies in spite of increased arterial perfusion pressures; the cause is not certain but it is probably due to increased cerebral arterial tone.

For fainting to occur consistently, both hypotension and an adjunct factor are necessary. For example, a moderate hemorrhage (10% of blood volume), a Valsalva maneuver or prolonged standing will all cause a decrease in cardiac output and a modest hypotension but none will, by itself ordinarily produce fainting. However, in all of them, a fainting tendency may be precipitated by an unnoticed hyperventilation.

While practically all individuals have one or two fainting episodes in their lifetime, there is a small but consistent fraction of the adult population, without apparent organic disease, which is prone to repeated fainting episodes. About 5% of blood donors, $e.g.$, have such fainting tendencies; reports indicate that such "fainters," compared to control subjects, experience a greater fall in arterial pressure and a greater decrease in alveolar P_{CO_2} to a standard 500-ml phlebotomy. Psychological tests further showed that the fainters also had a greater tendency toward hypochondriasis and depression than did control subjects; such studies suggest an interrelationship between psychic factors and hemodynamic response to stress which might account for the tendency toward circulatory collapse in these individuals. As described in Chapter 10, such psychogenic fainting may involve the depressor area of the hypothalamus.

REFERENCES

ABBOUD, F. M., D. D. HEISTAD, A. L. MARK, AND P. G. SCHMID: Reflex control of the peripheral circulation. *Prog. Cardiovasc. Dis.* 18:371, 1976.

FOX, I. J., W. P. CROWLEY, J. B. GRACE AND E. H. WOOD: Effects of the valsalva maneuver on blood flow in the thoracic aorta in man. *J. Appl. Physiol.* 21:1553, 1966.

FREY, M. A. B., AND R. A. KENNEY: Changes in left ventricular activity during apnea and face immersion. *Undersea Biomed. Res.* 4:27, 1977.

GAUER, O. N., AND H. L. THRON: Postural change in the circulation. In *Handbook of Physiology*, Section 2: *Circulation*, vol. III, ed. by W. F. Hamilton and P. Dow, p. 2409. Washington, D.C.: American Physiological Society, 1965.

HEISTAD, D. D., F. M. ABBOUD, AND J. W. ECKSTEIN: Vasoconstrictor response to simulated diving in man. *J. Appl. Physiol.* 25:542, 1968.

KLEIN, L. J., H. S. SALTZMAN, A. HEYMAN AND H. O. SICKER: Syncope induced by the Valsalva maneuver. *Am. J. Med.* 37:273, 1964.

LOGIC, J. R., S. A. JOHNSON, AND J. J. SMITH: Cardiovascular and hematologic responses to phlebotomy in blood donors. *Transfusion* 3:83, 1963.

MCHENRY, L. C., J. F. FAZEKAS, AND J. F. SULLIVAN: Cerebral hemodynamics of syncope. *Am. J. Med. Sci.* 241:173, 1961.

RUETZ, P. D., S. A. JOHNSON, R. CALLAHAN, R. E. MEADE, AND J. J. SMITH: Fainting: A review of the mechanisms and a study in blood donors. *Medicine* 46:363, 1967.

RYAN, C., M. HOLLENBERG, D. B. HARVEY, AND R. GWYNN: Impaired parasympathetic responses in patients after myocardial infarction. *Am. J. Cardiol.* 37:1013, 1976.

SHARPEY-SCHAFER, E. P.: Effect of respiratory acts on the circulation. In *Handbook of Physiology*, Section 2: *Circulation*, vol. III, ed. by W. F. Hamilton and P. Dow, p. 1875. Washington, D.C.: American Physiological Society, 1965.

SMITH, J. J., M. L. BONIN, V. T. WIEDMEIER, J. H. KALBFLEISCH, AND D. J. McDERMOTT: Cardiovascular response of young men to diverse stresses. *Aerosp. Med.* 45:583, 1974.

TRISTANI, F. E., D. G. KAMPER, D. J. McDERMOTT, B. J. PETERS, AND J. J. SMITH: Alteration of postural and valsalva responses in coronary heart disease. *Am. J. Physiol.* 233:H694, 1977.

chapter 14

Pathophysiology: Ischemic Heart Disease and Congestive Heart Failure

CIRCULATORY PATHOPHYSIOLOGY—GENERAL

The next two chapters are intended to show in a limited sense, how disease may alter the physiology and how the disordered state often helps us to better understand the normal. An understanding of the pathophysiology often requires basic investigation as well as observation of the patient. Dr. Carl J. Wiggers, one of our truly great cardiovascular physiologists, was fond of saying that the mistakes of nature, *i.e.*, disease, can best be solved by shuttling the problems back and

254

forth between the clinic and the experimental laboratory. In these chapters, in which we present capsule descriptions of four of the more common cardiovascular diseases, we have, therefore, also included accounts of basic studies and animal experiments insofar as they relate to the disease process.

In the following discussions of pathophysiology, the term *anoxia* refers to a complete absence of an oxygen supply, local or general. *Hypoxia* denotes a state of reduced oxygen supply. *Ischemia* is a condition of reduced perfusion of blood, local or general. Hypoxia (or anoxia) is classically subdivided into four types, *i.e.*, hypoxic, anemic, stagnant and histotoxic.

Hypoxic hypoxia is a condition in which there is a reduction of Po_2 of arterial blood; this may be caused by an inadequate partial pressure of oxygen in inspired air (*e.g.*, by ascent to altitude), by hypoventilation, or by lung disease in which there is an inadequate transfer of oxygen from the alveoli to the pulmonary capillary blood. *Anemic hypoxia* is the result of an inadequate amount of hemoglobin to carry the oxygen, *i.e.*, a reduced oxygen carrying capacity, such as may occur in anemia or carbon monoxide poisoning. *Stagnant hypoxia* is a condition in which blood flow is so diminished that insufficient oxygen is delivered to the tissues despite a normal blood Po_2 and normal hemoglobin concentration; this commonly occurs in low-flow states such as circulatory shock or congestive heart failure.

In *histotoxic hypoxia*, both the oxygen carrying capacity of blood and the tissue perfusion are adequate but the oxygen is denied to the cells because of the presence of a toxic agent. This may occur as a result of cyanide poisoning in which cellular hypoxia is produced through paralysis of the electron transfer function of cytochrome oxidase. *Cyanosis* is a bluish discoloration of the tissues due to reduced hemoglobin. The discoloration becomes evident particularly in the nail beds of the fingers, lips and mucous membranes when the blood concentration of reduced hemoglobin exceeds 5 g/dl; it commonly accompanies states of severe heart failure and advanced lung disease.

ISCHEMIC HEART DISEASE (IHD)

Since not all coronary artery disease results in cardiac ischemia and since cardiac ischemia can result from non-coronary diseases, ischemic heart disease (IHD) is the preferable term to designate changes occurring in the myocardium from reduction of blood flow (ischemia) or reduction of oxygen supply (hypoxia). IHD is the leading single cause of mortality in the western world and in the United States alone accounts for over 600,000 deaths annually; obviously it is a clinical and social problem of the highest magnitude. It primarily affects males in their forties or older. Unfortunately the disease is usually insidious and "silent" in the sense that symptoms appear late and early diagnosis is at present a virtual impossibility.

The primary factor contributing to IHD is coronary arteriosclerosis, a general term for thickening and hardening of the arterial wall. Atherosclerosis, the most prevalent type of arteriosclerosis, is the basic lesion, not only in coronary heart disease but in cerebrovascular disease and most renal and peripheral vascular diseases as well. Atheroslcerosis apparently begins with the deposition of cholesterol beneath the arterial intima; why the process accelerates in IHD is not certain but appears to be related to hyperlipidemia, *i.e.*, increased triglyceride and low density lipoprotein but most importantly, increased cholesterol levels of plasma. Hypercholesteremia, hypertension and cigarette smoking have been established as major risk factors in coronary artery disease; diabetes mellitus, obesity, physical inactivity, emotional stress and a positive family history of atherosclerosis are additional contributing factors. The tendency of hyperlipidémic subjects to coronary disease is illustrated in Figure 14-1.

Only when the arteriosclerotic process has progressed sufficiently to produce at least a 70% luminal narrowing of one or more of the three primary coronary arteries (or one of their larger branches) is the disease apt to manifest symptoms. The two main clinical forms of ischemic heart disease are angina pectoris and myocardial infarction. Both are characterized by precordial chest pains which may radiate to the left shoulder, arm and back. During periods of angina, the ECG may show ST and T wave changes and in myocardial infarction, abnormal Q waves.

The diagnosis of IHD is made primarily on the basis of a history of angina or myocardial infarction and confirmed by exercise stress test (Chapter 12), cardiac catheterization and angiography. In the latter procedure, the cardiac chambers, particularly the left ventricle, are filled with a radioopaque dye (ventriculography) during which motion pictures are taken of the fluoroscopy and later reviewed. From these films are determined end-diastolic volume (EDV), end-systolic volume

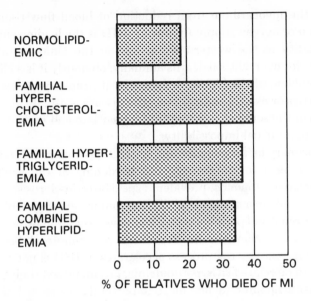

Figure 14-1. Predisposition of familial hyperlipidemic subjects to myocardial infarct (MI). MI death rates in adult, first degree relatives of hyperlipidemic MI patients were twice as high as relatives of normolipidemic patients. (From J. L. Goldstein, *The Myocardium: Failure and Infarction.* New York: HP Publishing Co., 1974.)

(ESV), ejection fraction (EF) and, very importantly, any defects in ventricular wall motion such as akinesia (defective contraction) or asynergy (non-uniform contraction); these defects might indicate a previous infarction. Finally, dye is injected directly into the coronary arteries so that any obstructive lesions may be visualized (arteriography).

Angina Pectoris

Angina pectoris is a condition featured by attacks of sudden substernal pain which may be described as "sharp" or "burning" or as a "tightness"; it may last several minutes and is the result of a transient, reversible, myocardial ischemia. The chest pain—sometimes severe— is associated with a temporary reduction of cardiac output, stroke volume and ventricular contractility. It may be accompanied by dyspnea (shortness of breath) or other signs of early heart failure. Angina pectoris is the result of a temporary disparity between myocardial oxygen demand and supply and is classically associated with the clinical sequence of "exertion-pain" and "rest-relief." Prompt cessation of the pain usually follows administration of nitrites.

Angina may be induced by exertion, emotional stress, increase in heart rate (pacing tachycardia) or by catecholamine infusion. However, in some patients the attack may develop without any evident prior physical or emotional strain or other apparent inciting cause. Patients with angina may remain "stable" for many years with only an occasional attack; on the other hand the condition may become progressive so that the attacks will become increasingly severe. While most angina patients have evidence of narrowing of the coronary arteries, a small percentage have, on angiography, anatomically normal coronary arteries. In such cases, it is thought that either the patient has disease of the smaller vessels (which are difficult to visualize) or that coronary arterial spasm is responsible for the myocardial ischemia. In any event, angina pectoris patients are more prone than normal subjects to an eventual myocardial infarct.

Myocardial Infarction

MI is a sudden irreversible, ischemic injury due to coronary arterial narrowing or occlusion with sustained damage to a segment of the myocardium; it is associated with electrocardiographic, metabolic and hemodynamic changes which depend on the size and location of the ischemic area. If the SA or AV nodes or a vital part of the conduction apparatus is affected, bradycardia, arrhythmia or conduction defects such as AV block may result. If as much as 20 or 25% of the left ventricular mass ceases to contract, there is usually hemodynamic evidence of left ventricular failure. Involvement of 40% or more results in severe pump failure with cardiogenic shock or death.

It is thought that complete obstruction is initiated at the damaged inner surface of an already partially occluded vessel, probably by accumulation of fibrin or platelets at the site. The exact sequence of events, however, is not certain and some investigators believe that the thrombosis actually occurs after the infarct rather than preceding it.

IHD takes an enormous toll of mortality and morbidity with a high incidence of sudden death in individuals completely unaware of their coronary disease. The increasing therapeutic capabilities which could now be applied if the existence of the disease were known make it abundantly clear that one of the great deficiencies in modern preventive medicine is the lack of an adequate method for the early diagnosis of ischemic heart disease.

Metabolic Changes and Coronary Blood Flow

Experimental studies have shown that if oxygen is cut off or perfusion is stopped in an isolated ventricle or working heart, depression of myocardial contractility begins within 15 seconds. Tissue Po_2 decreases and when it falls below 5 mm Hg, high energy phosphate concentration (mainly creatine phosphate) decreases and lactate concentration and glycolytic activity is increased. There is intracellular edema and swelling of sarcoplasmic reticulum and mitochondria and within 1 to 2 hours after hypoxia or ischemia the changes become irreversible.

However, ischemia and hypoxia produce very different biochemical and pathological effects. During ischemia, the acid products of glycolysis are not washed out, lactic acid concentration rises and intracellular pH falls rapidly. Both oxidative metabolic and anaerobic production of ATP are diminished and eventually glycolysis is inhibited and lactate production falls off. This lower glycolytic flux probably results from the acidotic inhibition of phosphofructokinase (PFK), a key enzyme in the glycolytic chain.

Normally lactate is taken up by the heart and oxidized so that the coronary arterial concentration exceeds the coronary venous concentration. With the acceleration of glycolysis in hypoxia and ischemia, this lactate gradient is reversed. From the infarcted myocardium there is an increased output of lactate as well as a release of certain enzymes such as glutamic oxalacetic transaminase (GOT), creatinine phosphokinase (CPK) and lactic dehydrogenase (LDH). The increase in serum concentration of these enzymes and their time course have proved diagnostically useful in MI.

Effect on Ventricular Contractility

As mentioned in Chapter 11, the greater net perfusion pressure to epicardial coronary vessels is generally offset by the greater metabolic vasodilation (autoregulation) in the subendocardial vessels. In the presence of restricted coronary blood flow and hypotension, coronary autoregulation declines and the subendocardium is further underperfused so that necrosis of subendocardium is much more common than that of the subepicardium. Following coronary occlusion, contractility of the epicardium is better preserved than the endocardium, apparently as a manifestation of this preferential perfusion of the outer wall.

After severe hypoxia or ischemia, the deterioration of myocardial function is abrupt and profound. In the early ischemic state, this functional decline occurs while high energy phosphate is still present in adequate amounts, so the latter does not appear to be the critical initiating factor. In their excellent review of the contractile mechanisms of the heart, Braunwald, Ross and Sonnenblick (1976) have pointed out that metabolic, electrical and contractile activities cease as necrosis develops and that the myocardial changes are generally permanent with eventual scar formation. The critical factors in the prognosis are the size of the infarct, the ability to limit its spread, the general condition of the heart and the assistance that can be rendered to the uninvolved myocardium.

Experimental ischemia of cardiac muscle usually results in a decrease or loss of contractile power with reduced contraction in the adjacent or marginal zones. In the uninvolved areas there are increased systolic, diastolic and stroke volume excursions as these segments assume a greater share of the contractile burden (Fig. 14-2).

If more than about 25% of myocardial mass is involved, there is usually a decrease in left ventricular stroke volume, stroke work and V_{max}. There is also an increase in ventricular EDV and EDP and a decrease in ventricular EF. With the loss of contractile power, the center of the ischemic zone may become immobile and, at first, bulges passively during ventricular systole, thus exhibiting "paradoxical" motion or dyskinesis.

However, shortly after the coronary occlusion, cellular swelling, edema and fibrocellular infiltration take place so that now the infarcted, non-contracting myocardial segment becomes stiff and contributes to the rise in EDP. These changes may produce abnormalities in cardiac sounds and ventricular wall motion; accentuated presystolic sounds and large "a" waves become evident on the phonocardiogram and on the apex cardiogram. Because a part of the myocardium is not functioning, asynergy of the ventricular muscle may appear on the ventriculogram (Fig. 14-3).

At a later time in the postinfarct period, the systolic tension generated by the contracting myocardium may possibly stretch and even-

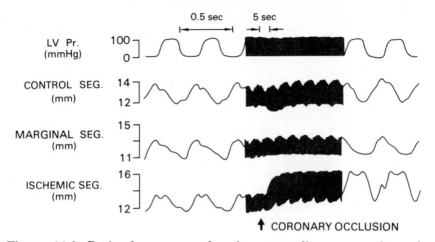

Figure 14-2. Regional responses of canine myocardium to experimental coronary occlusion. Occlusion was produced at the arrow; the degree of shortening (or lengthening) of muscle is indicated in the lower three tracings. Within 15 seconds after occlusion, the ischemic segment bulged and remained expanded both in systole and diastole. The marginal segment showed some increase in end-diastolic length and decrease in systolic shortening. The control non-ischemic segment shows an initial increased shortening with a later increase in end-diastolic length and degree of shortening, a compensatory response of the uninvolved muscle. The left ventricular pressure (*upper*) remained unchanged. (From P. Theroux, D. Franklin, J. Ross, Jr., and W. S. Kemper, *Circ. Res.* 35:896, 1974. By permission of the American Heart Association.)

tually disrupt and weaken the tissue of the non-contracting segment with accentuated bulging during systole and aneurysm formation. In accord with Laplace's law (Chapter 1), the wall stress will increase progressively and may further enlarge the ischemic zone.

General Hemodynamic Effects of MI

The result of a myocardial infarct on systemic hemodynamics is not always predictable; sometimes a systemic pressor and sometimes a depressor response results. Randall and others have pointed out that this variability may be due to cardiopulmonary baroceptors and specifically to the cardio-cardiac reflexes which are important in self-regulation of the heart. It has recently been shown, *e.g.*, that in the dog, ischemia of the inferoposterior myocardium will activate vagal

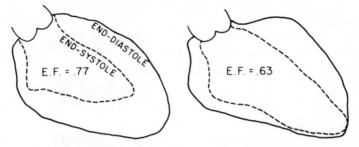

Figure 14-3. Left ventricular angiograms showing normal contraction pattern (*left*) and impaired contraction (*right*) because of hypokinesis of apical inferior area, with a fall in ejection fraction (EF). (From E. A. Amsterdam, R. R. Miller, D. H. Foley, and D. T. Mason, in *Peripheral Circulation,* ed. by R. Zelis. New York: Grune & Stratton, Inc. 1975.)

receptors in that area and induce a much more pronounced cardioinhibitory and vasodepressor response than a comparable anterior myocardial ischemia.

Another study involving MI patients within an hour of their attack showed that either vagal depressor or sympathetic pressor states may predominate. It seems evident, therefore, that in acute MI, there are not only direct hemodynamic changes resulting from the weakened myocardium but also important reflex responses arising from the activation of cardiopulmonary sensory receptors particularly in the myocardium. The nature of these hemodynamic reflex responses are importantly influenced by the site and extent of the infarct.

Patients who have recovered from an MI or who have chronic angina pectoris have shown altered circulatory responses to certain autonomic stresses. Recent reports have indicated that in such patients there was a lesser heart rate slowing during phase IV of the Valsalva test and a lesser vasoconstrictor response to upright tilt with a greater decline in systolic pressure. It is suspected that such changes in sympathetic and parasympathetic responses may be due to a decrease in sensitivity of arterial or cardiopulmonary baroceptors; however, the underlying cause is not known. Investigations are currently underway to explore the possibility that these altered autonomic reflexes may be useful as adjunctive tests for the diagnosis and characterization of IHD.

Treatment of IHD

Since the pathophysiological development of IHD is mainly the result of a disproportion between myocardial oxygen demand and supply, treatment is primarily aimed at favorable redressing of this balance. Because the oxygen extraction ratio is normally very high in the coronary bed, any increase in oxygen delivery must be achieved mainly by increased perfusion.

Nitroglycerin and other nitrites, which are widely used to relieve anginal attacks, reduce $M\dot{V}o_2$ by reducing venous tone and peripheral resistance and, therefore, serve to reduce preload, afterload and arterial pressure. The decreased LVEDV and myocardial tension override the disadvantages of the tachycardia, increased cardiac contractility and the consequent increased oxygen demand which result from the baroceptor response to the induced hypotension. The direct coronary dilator action of the nitrites is a secondary and less important one compared to the above effects.

Beta-adrenergic Blockade. As induced, *e.g.*, by propranolol, beta-adrenergic blockade exerts a beneficial effect by minimizing the increase in heart rate and myocardial contractility which may occur during stress. Its effectiveness in IHD is indicated by the fact that many patients receiving this drug will have less release of myocardial lactate during activity. This medication is, however, contraindicated in heart failure since it would deprive the myocardium of the compensatory sympathetic stimulation which is a support of the weakened muscle in failure.

Direct Myocardial Revascularization. The surgical construction of a bypass venous graft around the obstructed vessel is done in certain cases to reduce pain, alleviate anginal symptoms and preserve the myocardium. It is also reported to increase ventricular performance and contractility. For treatment of left main coronary artery occlusion, surgical treatment seems established. However, the relative effectiveness of medical *versus* surgical treatment of one or two vessel coronary artery disease is still an unsettled question.

Cardiac Rehabilitation. The long-term treatment of cardiac patients during their recovery from MI or cardiac surgery requires a careful, coordinated, interdisciplinary effort involving not only physicians and nurses but physical therapists and other members of the medical team. This very important phase of treatment aims at restoration of the patient's physical condition through systematic exercise training, diet and reduction of stress. It also has the objective of maintaining a favorable social and psychological environment through proper counseling and, if possible, an early return to work with the help of occupational counseling and vocational rehabilitation. The majority of patients who follow such a rehabilitation regimen after an MI are greatly benefitted by improved working capacity, greater emotional stability and a distinctly more productive and satisfying life.

CONGESTIVE HEART FAILURE

Etiology

Congestive failure is a condition in which the heart is unable to pump blood at a rate commensurate with systemic metabolic requirements. It is not a single disease but rather a symptom complex with many causes. Although there is still a considerable knowledge gap, our understanding of the pathophysiology of this disorder has been greatly advanced in recent years. Some of these developments will be discussed in outline form in this section.

The basic cause of the cardiac output deficiency in congestive failure may be *cardiac* or *extracardiac*. The *cardiac* disturbance may be (a) a myocardial contractile failure due to ischemic heart disease, myocarditis or cardiomyopathy (degeneration of the myocardium), or (b) a disorder which prevents proper filling or emptying of the heart such as a valvular stenosis, valvular regurgitation or pericardial disease. *Extracardiac* disorders which may cause congestive failure are high-pressure overloads such as hypertension, or high-output overloads such as renal failure, anemia, AV fistula or thyrotoxicosis. The apparent paradox of a heart failing because of increased output is the result of myocardial work demands in excess of coronary flow capabilities.

From a therapeutic standpoint it would be important to know whether the failure is due to an extracardiac, valvular or pericardial disorder, which may be remediable, in contrast to a basic myocardial, contractile weakness, which is not.

Hemodynamic Mechanisms in Development of Congestive Failure

Controversy has long centered on the question of whether this disorder was primarily a *backward cardiac failure;* in this case the decreased ventricular output and the rising ventricular EDP produced, through retrograde action, increased venous and capillary pressures. The resulting fluid transudation into the tissue spaces contracts the plasma volume which presumably "signals" an increase in tubular reabsorption of sodium and water. It was theorized that this combination of heightened capillary pressure and renal "hyperfunction" resulted in pulmonary and peripheral congestion and edema.

In contrast, the *forward-failure theory* held that the symptoms and signs stemmed from an inadequate left ventricular output with a reduction of renal perfusion pressure and glomerular filtration, and as a consequence, increased sodium and water reabsorption through the renin-angiotensin-aldosterone mechanism. Because it is now known that both mechanisms operate to varying degrees, this classification is not currently useful and has been generally abandoned.

The signs and symptoms of the failure are ascribable to three main hemodynamic changes, *i.e., decreased cardiac output* with hypoperfusion of the peripheral bed, *increased left atrial pressure* with resulting pulmonary congestion and *increased right atrial pressure* with resultant systemic and splanchnic congestion.

The *decrease in cardiac output* is primarily responsible for the ↓C.O. limitation of physical activity, the renal hypoperfusion, the sodium and water retention and the chronic fatigue which is characteristic of this condition; fatigue may precede the other symptoms by many months. The *increased left atrial pressure,* the aftermath of the ↑ P_La increased LVEDV and LVEDP, results in increased size of the atrium, increased pulmonary venous and capillary pressure, pulmonary congestion and edema and, if continued, decrease in pulmonary airspace and pulmonary compliance with resultant dyspnea and orthopnea.

Increased Right Atrial Pressure. This will produce comparable changes in the systemic circulation, *i.e.,* increased volume and pressure in the vena cavae, peripheral veins and capillaries with peripheral edema particularly of the feet and ankles. There is also increased hepatic venous pressure with hepatic congestion and, if continued, liver dysfunction and intraperitoneal accumulation of fluid (ascites). Increased right atrial pressure may develop from pulmonic valve stenosis or regurgitation but more commonly is a backward extension of increased left atrial pressure and pulmonary venous congestion.

In some cases, only one or two of these hemodynamic changes may occur, but all three frequently develop in the same patient. Signs and symptoms may vary considerably depending on the severity and rate of development of the underlying disorder. As mentioned earlier, a myocardial infarct involving over 40% of the myocardium will probably cause a hemodynamic collapse and cardiogenic shock. On the other hand, a patient may, from a lesser lesion, be in "compensated failure" for many years without severe disability until another infarct, infection or other complication may intensify the condition.

Pathophysiological and Compensatory Changes in Congestive Failure

The most important manifestations of congestive failure are those involving (a) the myocardium, (b) fluid balance, (c) bioenergetics, and (d) the peripheral circulation. These will be discussed in the following sections.

Myocardial Failure and Compensatory Responses

In congestive failure, both clinical and experimental, there is usually a deficit in ventricular contractility as evidenced by depressed length-tension and ventricular function curves (Fig. 14-4, *curve c*).

In addition the myocardium usually shows a decreased force-velocity curve, thus clearly indicating inotropic inadequacy of the myocardium. This contractile defect may arise from a primary myocardial lesion such as MI or from a secondary ischemia resulting from a ventricular pressure or output overload.

The *ejection fraction* (EF), which is an important measure in heart failure, is positively correlated with the cardiac index. With the decline in left ventricular performance, the EF decreases from its normal value of about 60 or 70% and in severe failure may be as low as 10 to 20%.

The two compensatory mechanisms available to improve myocardial performance, *i.e.,* the *Starling effect* and the *sympathetic inotropic effect* (Chapter 6) are both activated in congestive failure; in addition, *ventricular volume and hypertrophy* changes also occur. These adaptions are discussed in the following.

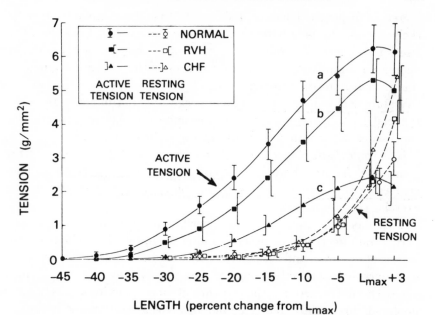

Figure 14-4. Length-tension curves for normal (○), hypertrophied (□) and failing (△) ventricular muscle in the cat. Lower curves show resting, passive tension and upper curves show peak contractile tension. Tension is corrected for cross-sectional area. In heart failure, maximum tension is clearly depressed but in hypertrophied muscle, depression is borderline. (From J. F. Spann, R. A. Buccino, E. H. Sonnenblick, and E. Braunwald, *Circ. Res.* 21:341, 1967. By permission of the American Heart Association, Inc.)

A. The Starling Effect. The decrease in cardiac output, aided by the increased sodium and water retention (discussed below), leads to progressive elevation of EDV and EDP. This increased diastolic stretch results in increased ventricular performance so long as the ventricle functions on the rising portion of the length-tension curve (Fig. 14-4, *curve c*). However, this improved ventricular performance is achieved at the price of pulmonary congestion in the case of the left ventricle, and systemic venous congestion in the case of the right.

Increased emphasis has been given recently to another effect of the increased EDV, namely the adverse influence of heightened EDV on ventricular diastolic compliance and the effect of the latter on the hemodynamics of congestive failure.

It will be noted in Figure 14-4 that as the ventricle fills and EDV and resting tension increase, the tension/length ratio, or stiffness, increases disproportionately. This means that the compliance (*i.e.*, its reciprocal or the length/tension ratio) decreases sharply as the EDV rises. This decreased compliance, coupled in the case of MI with the decreased compliance incident to stiffening of the ischemic segment of the myocardium (mentioned earlier) tends to perpetuate the congestive state. Some investigators have suggested that in some cases the reduced diastolic compliance may be as important a factor in producing congestion as the impaired ventricular systolic contractility.

B. Sympathetic Inotropic Effect—Myocardial Response. During congestive failure, there is augmented sympathetic activity and increased concentration of plasma norepinephrine at rest and during exercise (Fig. 14-5).

This has both myocardial and peripheral circulatory effects; the peripheral effects will be described later in this section. The resultant increase in force and velocity of myocardial contraction exerts a considerable functional support for the heart. However, with continued sympathetic overactivity, the myocardial catecholamine stores become depleted, due mainly to a reduction of myocardial tyrosine hydroxylase, which is the rate-limiting step for the conversion of tyrosine to norepinephrine. This depletion is apparently not involved however, in the pathogenesis of failure; it may be that the residual catecholamines from the adrenal medulla and other sources remain effective because of the *de facto* denervation of the myocardium and the consequent hypersensitivity response to catechols (Chapter 9).

C. Ventricular Volume and Hypertrophy. If a cardiac chamber is subjected to continued distension from an increased preload or afterload stress, its internal capacity will increase; if it is required to consistently produce increased muscular work, either by a volume or pressure overload, it will hypertrophy, *i.e.*, the number of sarcomeres will increase, the wall becomes thicker and the muscle will increase in mass. Pressure work, *e.g.*, in hypertension, is particularly effective in producing such hypertrophy. In most cases, such as occurs physiologically in the endurance athlete and pathologically in congestive failure, there is an increase in both ventricular volume and mass. But changes in myocardial volume and mass are different phenomena and exert independent effects.

As the left ventricular chamber enlarges during early failure, it assumes a more spherical shape and the increased EDV, as described

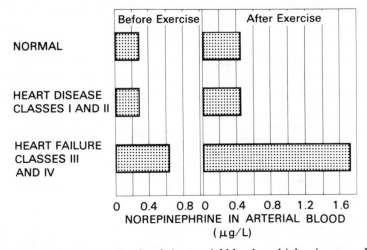

Figure 14-5. Norepinephrine levels in arterial blood are higher in severe heart failure patients (class III and IV) at rest and after exercise than in normal subjects or in patients with milder heart failure (I and II). (From E. Braunwald, *The Myocardium: Failure and Infarction.* New York: HP Publishing Co., 1974.)

above, has a compensatory, supportive action. However, a continued EDV increase eventually becomes self-defeating because in an expanding, more spherical ventricle, the total force required for an equivalent systolic ejection against a comparable afterload will also increase as the radius increases (Laplace's law). Since myocardial $\dot{V}o_2$ is closely correlated with the ventricular wall stress which generates the cardiac force (Chapter 11), the oxygen demand becomes disproportionately greater than the stroke work produced and the process becomes inefficient. This effect on wall stress is only partially offset by the fact that at a larger ventricular size, a given fraction of circumferential shortening will result in a larger stroke volume.

Hypertrophy, *i.e.*, increased mass, is a compensatory mechanism which increases the force-generating capacity of the ventricle; the contractility of the hypertrophied muscle is only slightly less than that of normal muscle (Fig. 14-4, *curve b*). Thus both contractile load and wall tension are spread over a greater muscle mass. Hypertrophy, therefore, in conjunction with the Starling and sympathetic inotropic effects, helps to maintain overall circulatory compensation.

However, there is also a limit to this adaptive process, imposed mainly by an already borderline coronary perfusion pressure supplying a growing tissue mass. The net benefit will depend on the ability of a limited hypertrophy to establish compensation. Unfortunately, increased wall thickness will also decrease wall compliance and in the case of severe failure with an already decreased ventricular compliance, this effect may be intensified.

Clinical and experimental studies have shown that myocardial hypertrophy is at least to some extent, reversible. Left ventricular hypertrophy incident to aortic stenosis may significantly regress after valve replacement surgery. Right ventricular hypertrophy, induced in cats by a 24-week application of constricting pulmonary arterial bands, reverted to normal size after band removal. This suggests that such myocardial changes, especially if generated over a relatively short time span, are not necessarily permanent.

Fluid Balance in Congestive Failure

As cardiac output decreases in congestive failure, the reduced renal arterial hydrostatic pressure as well as the reflex renal vasoconstriction (described below) combine to reduce renal blood flow, particularly in the outer renal cortex. There results a reduction in glomerular filtration rate which leads to salt and water retention and eventually, if continued, to edema. The mechanism resembles the response to hemorrhage described in Chapter 13; the reduced renal blood flow leads to the liberation of renin, the elaboration of angiotensin II and ultimately to the production of aldosterone by the zona glomerulosa of the adrenal cortex.

The hepatic dysfunction which accompanies severe congestive failure is responsible for a reduced catabolism of aldosterone so that aldosterone plasma levels are higher and more sustained, thus accentuating the fluid retention. Renal venous congestion plays a variable but generally limited role in the fluid balance disturbance.

Thus patients with congestive failure usually have increased blood volume, interstitial fluid volume and increased total body sodium levels; however, this may be associated with normal or even decreased serum Na^+ concentrations. Increased physical activity, because it causes increased sympathetic stimulation and heightened plasma norepinephrine, will result in further lowering of renal blood flow and the glomerular filtration rate and will increase the salt and water retention. Thus, during the decompensated phase of congestive failure, rest and restricted activity are an important part of therapy.

Bioenergetics of Congestive Heart Failure

The biochemical changes accompanying muscle contraction may be divided into three sequential processes: energy production or the conversion of substrates to high energy phosphates; energy utilization, *i.e.*, the translation of high energy phosphates to contractile activity; and excitation-contraction coupling, the mechanism by which the myocardial action potential results in calcium movement, which in turn mediates the contraction and relaxation (Chapter 6).

Studies have shown that even in severe failure, mitochondrial function is not disturbed so that energy production appears adequate. ATP is converted to ADP primarily during the interaction of myosin and actin to produce shortening; the rate of this reaction correlates well with contractility. It has been shown that there is a deficiency in the myofibrillar-ATPase system in severe failure and some reduction of function in myocardial hypertrophy without failure, but the full implications of these defects are not yet known.

In some types of congestive failure, the ATP-dependent calcium pump of the isolated sarcoplasmic reticulum is defective. Both the amount and the rate at which calcium is pumped into the sarcoplasmic reticulum are deficient and with the development of hypertrophy, the content of sarcoplasmic reticulum per muscle unit is reduced; thus there may be a dilution of sarcoplasmic reticulum incident to the hypertrophy process itself. It is, therefore, evident that biochemical defects do exist in the failing muscle, but which are the critical ones is not yet known.

Peripheral Circulation in Congestive Failure

There is in congestive failure a significant redistribution of left ventricular output, which, like hypervolemia, is an important compensatory mechanism (Fig. 14-6).

This redistribution is mainly the result of sympathetic vasoconstriction which diverts the renal and cutaneous portions of an already reduced cardiac output to the more critical cerebral and coronary beds. This occurs even at rest but is intensified in the presence of exercise, fever or other stresses.

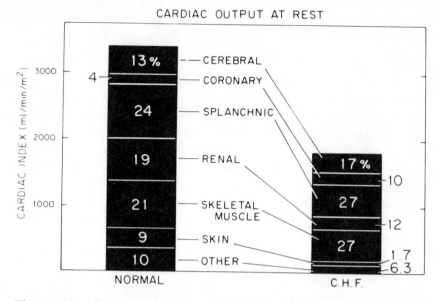

Figure 14-6. Decrease in cardiac index (CI) and alteration in fractional distribution of CI in congestive failure patients (CHF). (From A. C. Hseih, *The Peripheral Circulation,* ed. by R. Zelis. New York: Grune & Stratton Inc., 1975.)

There is a general increased tone of peripheral arteries and veins and with only modest physical activity, a marked vasoconstriction of mesenteric and renal vascular beds as well. The heightened tone of the peripheral vessels is partially due to an increased infiltration of sodium and water into the arterial walls. The net result is a reduced ability of the vessels to dilate with increased activity so that oxygen extraction is limited (Fig. 14-7). Exercise or increased metabolic states will, therefore, produce lactic acidemia and an inability to dissipate heat. Consequently, the heart failure patient frequently has a heat intolerance.

The cause of the heightened sympathetic activity is not certain but is probably due, at least in part, to a lessened arterial baroceptor stimulation secondary to a decrease in arterial pressure. Increased cardiopulmonary receptor activity from the affected heart and lungs and increased chemoreceptor stimulation from the elevated Pco_2 and lowered pH may also contribute to sympathetic activation. Heart

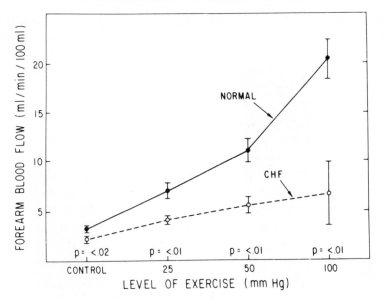

Figure 14-7. Forearm blood flow in congestive heart failure patients (CHF) increased less during handgrip exercise than that of normal subjects at all exercise levels showing inability of peripheral vessels to dilate properly to metabolic stimulus. (From A. C. Hseih, *The Peripheral Circulation,* ed. by R. Zelis. New York: Grune & Stratton Inc., 1975.)

failure is also associated with a marked deficiency of parasympathetic function as shown, *e.g.,* by a marked reduction of the bradycardic reflex response to both arterial hypertension and to the pressure overshoot phase of the Valsalva test.

As previously mentioned, the decreased ability to alter peripheral blood flow is of considerable functional significance to heart failure patients. Equally disadvantageous is the reduced ability to alter heart rate. Since these patients already have severe limitations in their ability to adjust stroke volume, the added rate limitation is an appreciable further handicap in meeting cardiac output needs.

Treatment of Congestive Failure

Therapy will depend on the severity and rate of development of the disease and will be directed first of all toward the specific cause of the failure. The treatment of the congestive failure itself usually has three objectives: (a) reduction of cardiac work load, (b) enhancement of cardiac contractility and (c) control of excessive fluid retention.

Reduction of Cardiac Work. This is done mainly by reducing afterload through rest, by minimizing physical and emotional stress, and sometimes through modest doses of nitroprusside and nitroglycerin. The latter agents reduce peripheral vessel resistance and preload, thereby reducing ventricular EDP and myocardial O_2 demands while increasing stroke volume. The objective is to bring this about with a minimal reduction in aortic pressure. In attempting to manipulate aortic pressure, a balance must be struck between a relatively low value to reduce afterload and cardiac work while maintaining a sufficiently high level to insure reasonable perfusion of the coronary bed and peripheral tissues. As previously mentioned, the autoregulatory capacity of the coronary bed is often compromised in heart failure so that flow is more directly dependent on perfusion pressure.

Glycosides. Digitalis and other glycosides have the fortuitous property of producing a more effective positive inotropic action in the failing than in the normal heart; this is probably due to a combination of its direct myocardial effect with an arteriolar and venular dilation action. In severe failure, morphine is effective in relieving dyspnea, probably by reducing sympathetic tone which results in a vasodilator and venodilator action; this increases venous capacitance and lessens preload. The depressant effect of morphine on the cerebral cortex also assists in reducing the perception of dyspnea.

In some cases, the above forms of treatment will also relieve fluid retention. If not, more specific therapy is used in the form of (a) *thiazide diuretics* which reduce tubular reabsorption of sodium and thus increase its excretion, or (b) agents such as furosemide or aldactone: (the latter because of its aldosterone-antagonist activity), which also exert powerful diuretic action.

Therapy must be carefully controlled. Although it is a pathological condition, hypervolemia is a compensatory change with a purpose. Rapid loss of fluid without improved cardiac performance might trade the edema for the increased fatigue of inadequate cardiac output. Overzealous use of diuretics with resultant hypovolemia must be particularly avoided.

REFERENCES

Ischemic Heart Disease

AMSTERDAM, E. A., R. R. MILLER, D. H. FOLEY, AND D. T. MASON: Pathophysiology and treatment of coronary artery disease. In *Peripheral Circulation,* ed. by R. Zelis. New York: Grune & Stratton Inc., 1975.

BLANKENHORN, D. H.: Reversibility of latent atherosclerosis. *Mod. Concepts Cardiovasc. Dis.* 47:79, 1978.

BOSNJAK, Z. J., E. J. ZUPERKU, R. L. COON, AND J. P. KAMPINE: Acute coronary artery occlusion and cardiac sympathetic afferent nerve activity. *Proc. Soc. Exp. Biol.* 161:38, 1979.

BRAUNWALD, E. A., J. ROSS, AND E. H. SONNENBLICK: *Mechanisms of Contraction of the Normal and Failing Heart,* 2nd ed., Boston: Little, Brown and Co., 1976.

BROOKS, H., R. HOLLAND, AND J. AL SADIR: Right ventricular performance during ischemia: An anatomic and hemodynamic analysis. *Am. J. Physiol.* 233:H500, 1978.

FREDERICKSON, D. S.: Atherosclerosis and other forms of arteriosclerosis. In *Principles of Internal Medicine,* 7th ed., ed. by M. M. Wintrobe. New York: McGraw-Hill Book Co., 1974.

GOLDSTEIN, R. E., G. D. BESIER, M. STAMPFER, AND J. E. EPSTEIN: Impairment of autonomically mediated heart rate control in patients with cardiac dysfunction. *Circ. Res.* 36:571–578, 1975.

HERMAN, M. V., AND R. GORLIN: Pathophysiology of ischemic heart disease. In *Clinical Cardiovascular Physiology,* ed. by H. J. Levine. New York: Grune & Stratton, Inc., 1976.

JAMES, T. N.: *Anatomy of the Coronary Arteries.* New York: Hoeber Medical Division, Harper & Row, Publishers, Inc., 1961.

PANTRIDGE, J. F., S. W. WEBB, A. A. J. ADGEY, AND J. S. GEDDES: The first hour after the onset of acute myocardial infarction. *Progress in Cardiology,* Chap. 5, pp. 173–188, 1974.

RANDALL, W. C.: *Neural Regulation of the Heart.* New York: Oxford University Press, 1977.

THAMES, M. D., H. S. KLOPFENSTEIN, F. W. ABBOUD, A. L. MARK, AND J. L. WALTER: Preferential distribution of inhibitory cardiac receptors with vagal afferents to the infero-posterior wall of the left ventricle activated during coronary occlusion in the dog. *Circ. Res.* 43:512–519, 1978.

TRISTANI, F. E., D. G. KAMPER, D. J. McDERMOTT, B. S. PETERS, AND J. J. SMITH: Alteration of postural and Valsalva responses in coronary heart disease. *Am. J. Physiol.* 233:H694–H699, 1977.

Congestive Heart Failure

BRAUNWALD, E., J. ROSS, AND E. H. SONNENBLICK: *Mechanisms of Contraction of the Normal and Failing Heart,* 2nd ed., Boston: Little, Brown and Co., 1976.

BRAUNWALD, E.: Heart failure. In *Principles of Internal Medicine,* 8th ed. New York: McGraw-Hill Book Co., 1977.

BRENNER, B. M., AND F. C. RECTOR: *The Kidney.* Philadelphia: W. B. Saunders & Co., 1976.

KIRK, E. S., C. W. URSCHEL, AND E. H. SONNENBLICK: Problems in cardiac performance: regulation of coronary blood flow and physiology of heart failure. *MTP International Review of Science,* ed. by A. C. Guyton and C. F. Jones. Baltimore: University Park Press, 1974.

LEVINE, H. J.: Congestive heart failure. In *Clinical Cardiovascular Physiology,* ed. by H. J. Levine. New York: Grune & Stratton Inc., 1976.

LEVINE, H. J., AND W. H. GAASCH: Diastolic compliance of the left ventricle. *Mod. Concepts Cardiovasc. Dis.,* 47:95–102, 1978.

MASON, D. T., R. ZELIS, AND J. WIKMAN-COFFELT: Symposium on congestive heart failure. *Am. J. Cardiol.* 32:395, 1973.

ZELIS, R., AND J. LONGHURST: The circulation in congestive heart failure. In *The Peripheral Circulation,* ed. by R. Zelis. New York: Grune & Stratton Inc., 1975.

chapter 15

Pathophysiology: Hypertension and Circulatory Shock

HYPERTENSION

Definitions and Classification

About 20% of the adult population are afflicted with hypertension—the most common single disorder seen in the office of an internist. It is a major risk factor for coronary artery disease and a common cause of heart failure, kidney failure, stroke and blindness. As Pickering has pointed out, the designation of a single dividing line between normo-tension and hypertension is somewhat artificial. The diagnosis is usually based on repeated resting levels of $\geq$ 140/90 mm Hg in adults 18 to 49 years of age and $\geq$ 160/95 mm Hg in adults over 50 years of age. It is more common among males than females and far more common among blacks than whites. Diastolic hypertension is more frequent than systolic. Obesity is a strong predisposing factor and hypertension is 10 times more common in persons 20% or more overweight.

About 10% of adult hypertension is due to a specific, identifiable, cause and is termed *secondary hypertension.* The remaining 90%, in which the cause cannot be determined, is classified as primary or *essential hypertension* (EH). The latter develops more often between the ages of 35 to 50 years. Hypertension developing during infancy or childhood or after the age of 50 is often of the secondary variety.

There are multiple ways in which arterial blood pressure can be raised and for almost each pressor mechanism, there is a representative example of a clinical type of hypertension. Only EH and a few of the more common types of secondary hypertension will be considered in this chapter. Because of the close relationship of the kidney to hyper-tension, a few aspects of renal circulation will be reviewed at this point.

Renal Circulation

Functional Anatomy. From the renal artery, interlobar arteries ascend between the pyramids and divide into arcuate arteries which in turn subdivide into interlobular vessels and thence into thick-walled afferent arterioles. The latter supply the glomerular capillaries (Fig. 15-1, *left*). The shorter, thin-walled, efferent arterioles subdivide to form the peritubular capillary plexuses which surround the cortical convoluted tubules. The efferent arterioles from the juxtamedullary nephrons drain downward into vasa recta in the proximity of the loops of Henle before turning back upward to empty into cortical veins.

Near the glomerulus, the afferent arteriolar wall is thickened asym-metrically and contains small specialized juxtaglomerular (JG) cells which are thought to be the site of renin formation; the portion of the distal tubule lying adjacent to the JG cells forms a small cellular plaque called the macula densa, which together with the JG cells is

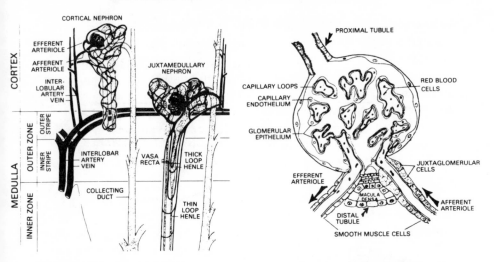

Figure 15-1. Renal circulation. *Left,* blood supply to cortical and juxtamedullary nephrons. *Right,* juxtaglomerular complex including JG cells and macula densa. (Reproduced with permission from R. F. Pitts, *Physiology of Kidney and Body Fluids,* 3rd ed. Chicago: Year Book Medical Publishers, Inc., 1974; A. Ham and T. Leeson, *Histology,* 4th ed. Philadelphia: J. B. Lippincott Co., 1961.)

termed the juxtaglomerular apparatus or JGA (Fig. 15-1, *right*). The JGA constitutes a regulatory system and increased renal sympathetic stimulation, reduced glomerular pressure and perhaps reduced sodium concentration of the tubular fluid will cause a release of renin into afferent arterioles and the general circulation.

General Regulation. As mentioned earlier (Chapter 9), the kidney, a highly vascular organ, receives about 20% of the total cardiac output but because of its modest oxygen consumption has a low oxygen extraction. It has been theorized that the JGA-renin mechanism may be involved in the high autoregulatory capability which is characteristic of the renal circulation (Chapter 9).

Increased sympathetic stimulation during exercise, emotion, postural change or hemorrhage will cause renin release *via* a beta-receptor mechanism. Renin is a determinant of aldosterone release and the renin-angiotensin-aldosterone sequence is important in the regulation of extracellular fluid volume and arterial pressure (Fig. 15-2).

In addition to the above mechanisms, vasopressin, the antidiuretic hormone (ADH) is also concerned with blood pressure and water

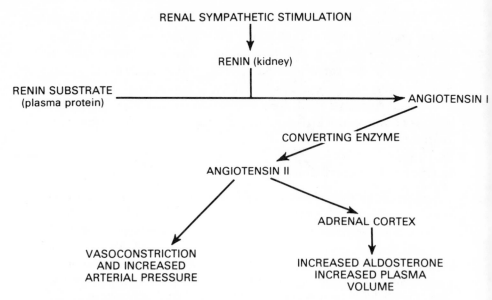

Figure 15-2. Renin-angiotensin-aldosterone mechanism. For maintenance of arterial blood pressure and extracellular fluid volume.

volume. Vasopressin, synthesized in the hypothalamus and stored in the posterior pituitary gland, increases water reabsorption from the distal tubules and thus expands plasma volume. Decreased atrial stretch, increased osmolality and emotional stress seem to be the main stimuli for its release. There is also some evidence that the renin-angiotensin system controls ADH release in part. In hypotensive states, the general vasoconstrictor action of vasopressin exerts a pressor effect adjunctive to that resulting from the arterial and cardiopulmonary baroceptor reflexes. The ADH system seems to act primarily in emergencies but its physiological role is still unclear. Diabetes insipidus, a rare disorder characterized by polyuria (excessive diuresis) and polydipsia (excessive thirst) is a vasopressin deficiency disease but usually with no primary blood pressure abnormality.

Intrarenal Blood Flow. Blood flow within the kidney is also affected by neurohumoral influences. Sympathetic vasoconstriction is more pronounced in the inner half of the renal cortex and as a consequence there is proportionately less flow to and less sodium excretion by the inner cortical nephrons than by the outer. However, most vasodilators, *e.g.,* histamine, dopamine and prostaglandins of the A and E series induce greater fractional flow to the inner cortex and medulla. It is thought that PGE_2, a particularly potent renal vasodilator which is synthesized in the renal medulla, thereby protects the renal parenchyma against the excessive salt and water conserving action of the renin-angiotensin system. It has been suggested that PGE_2 deficiency may play a role in the genesis of EH, but the evidence thus far is only fragmentary.

Secondary Hypertension

Renovascular Hypertension. Renal diseases are the most frequent cause of secondary hypertension and include two clinical entities, *renovascular hypertension,* a disease of the renal arteries, and *renal parenchymal hypertension.* While kidney disease and hypertension have long been clinically associated, the relation between the two was obscure until Goldblatt showed that persistent hypertension could be produced experimentally by constriction of the renal arteries. With the discovery of angiotensin and its synthesis, a possible relation of the renin-angiotensin mechanism to renal arterial hypertension began to emerge (Fig. 15-2).

Angiotensin II raises arterial pressure through its very potent vasoconstrictor action and also through stimulation of aldosterone secretion with the resultant sodium retention. However, it is evident that the mechanism of renovascular hypertension is complex since only about two thirds of these patients have elevated levels of plasma renin activity. Nevertheless the measurement of renin or angiotensin activity of the blood or a trial of an angiotensin antagonist are sometimes useful diagnostic screening procedures. Beta-adrenergic blockade can reduce renin activity and, therefore, is sometimes used in hypertension therapy.

Renal Parenchymal Hypertension. This occurs in a variety of acute and chronic renal parenchymal diseases such as pyelonephritis (inflammation of the renal pelvis) or chronic glomerulonephritis. It is thought that the underlying cause is a decreased renal perfusion due to inflammatory and fibrotic changes. However, peripheral plasma renin activity is elevated far less frequently than in renovascular hypertension. Aside from the renal ischemia, the hypertension has also been explained on the basis of an unidentified vasopressor substance, a prostaglandin deficiency or an ischemia due to increased sodium and water infiltration of the arteriolar walls with narrowing of the lumina.

Endocrine Hypertension. Clinically and experimentally, it is known that when about 70% of the kidney mass has been destroyed and fluid and sodium intake increased, a "volume-loading hypertension" will be produced. It is basically the sodium which is responsible, since a persistent hypertension will not result with only a water retention. Similar types of hypertension will result from a number of endocrine disorders such as *primary aldosteronism*, a condition due to an adrenal tumor with excessive aldosterone secretion and increased sodium reabsorption; there is frequently an associated muscle weakness due to potassium depletion.

Hypertension will also occur in *Cushing's syndrome* which is characterized by excessive secretion of glucocorticoids and sodium retention. Another cause of hypertension is *pheochromocytoma*, an adrenal medullary tumor in which there is increased secretion of epinephrine and norepinephrine associated with chronic peripheral vasoconstriction and myocardial hyperkinesis; in this disorder, heightened sympathetic tone rather than volume expansion is the main characteristic. *Mineralocorticoid hypertension* is characterized by low plasma levels of renin and aldosterone but elevated secretion of desoxycorticosterone (DOCA) or DOCA analogues, often associated with hypokalemia. In some of these patients, the administration of an aldosterone antagonist such as spironolactone will result in a loss of sodium and a lowering of the blood pressure.

Other Types of Hypertension. There are other varieties of hypertension in which the inciting cause is known but the mechanism is uncertain. These include hypertension due to drugs such as oral contraceptives or monoamine oxidase and those due to hypercalcemia and to the toxemia of pregnancy. Hypertension, primarily systolic in nature, can also be caused by coarctation of the aorta, hyperthyroidism and decreased distensibility of the aorta.

Essential Hypertension

Hemodynamic Changes. Hypertension is closely linked with the atherosclerotic process; with continued pressure elevation, the latter will be progressive regardless of the cause of the hypertension. Thus if unchecked, EH eventually leads to ischemic heart disease, cerebrovascular disorders or renal disease with uremia (accumulation of urea and other protein metabolites in the blood). In some cases, for unknown reasons, the process becomes accelerated (malignant hypertension).

As discussed in Chapter 2, increase in arterial pressure may result from increase of either cardiac output or peripheral vascular resistance or both. Increased peripheral vascular resistance (due to heightened vasoconstriction) is practically a universal accompaniment of clinical hypertension. However, patients with renovascular disease, coarctation of the aorta or labile (periodic) hypertension frequently have, in addition, increased cardiac output, heart rate and increased left ventricular ejection, *i.e.*, a tendency toward ventricular hyperkinesis. In contrast, patients with hypertension due to renal parenchymal disease, aldosteronism or Cushing's syndrome, *i.e.*, a volume-loading hypertension, are more apt to have a normal cardiac output associated with the elevated peripheral resistance and increased heart rate.

In EH and many other types of hypertension, increased cardiac output is often an early feature of the disease. Some investigators believe the increased output to be the critical initiator of the arteriosclerosis which then triggers the progression of the disease; later the cardiac output usually reverts to normal levels.

All forms of hypertension seem to be related to an increased heart rate which would of course not be expected in the presence of active arterial and cardiopulmonary baroceptor reflexes. Clinical and experimental studies have established the fact that these reflexes still moderate the pressure but have been "reset" at a higher baseline. But the basic cause of this dissociation of arterial pressure and heart rate is not known. Tachycardia is undoubtedly a significant facet of the pathophysiology and it is conceivable that the baroceptor reset may be one of the initial steps in the pathogenesis of the disease.

Changes in plasma volume are rather unique in hypertension and vary depending on clinical type. In renal parenchymal and most other forms of volume loading hypertension, there is a direct relationship between plasma volume and diastolic or mean arterial pressure (Fig. 15-3). This might be predicted from the venous return curves discussed in Chapter 7 in a situation in which peripheral resistance is normal or

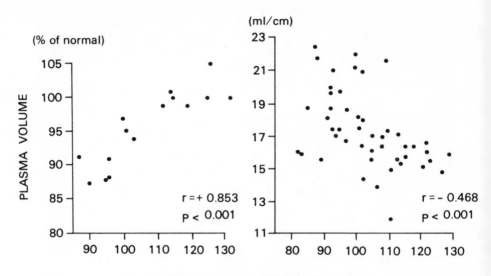

Figure 15-3. Variable relationship between plasma volume and diastolic pressure in different types of hypertension. *Left,* a positive correlation between plasma volume (noted as per cent of normal) and diastolic pressure in renal parenchymal (a volume-loading) type of hypertension. *Right,* a highly significant inverse correlation between plasma volume and diastolic pressure in essential hypertension. (From R. C. Tarazi, H. P. Dustan, E. D. Frohlich, R. W. Gifford, and G. C. Hoffman, *Arch. Int. Med.* 125:835, 1970. Copyright 1970, American Medical Association.)

increased. However, in many cases of EH, renovascular hypertension and pheochromocytoma, there is an inverse relationship between the diastolic pressure and plasma volume (Fig. 15-3); this is probably a reflection of the decrease in plasma volume usually associated with a heightened sympathetic tone and a consequent general decrease in vascular capacity.

As mentioned earlier, in renovascular and other types of hypertension associated with renal ischemia, elevated plasma renin levels would be expected. However, in some cases of early essential hypertension, there may also occur a rise in plasma renin activity, presumably because of heightened sympathetic activity or alteration in intrarenal hemodynamics. In primary aldosteronism and other forms of volume-loaded hypertension, the elevated plasma volume is often associated with a reduced plasma renin activity.

There are significant changes in autonomic responsiveness in hypertension. Baroreflex sensitivity is reduced in older individuals and in hypertensive patients; in the latter there is, in contrast to the usual situation (Chapter 10), a greater sensitivity to hypertensive rather than hypotensive stimuli, ostensibly an effort to limit further pressure elevation.

Reports indicate that during head-up tilt, borderline hypertensives have a significantly greater rise in diastolic pressure than normal subjects but that patients with advanced disease have a decline (orthostatic hypotension); the early orthostatic hypertension may reflect the increased plasma volume and ventricular hyperkinesis common at this stage. Hypertensive patients have also been found to respond to mental arithmetic and other stressful experiences with an exaggerated rise in blood pressure. Other investigators have reported the blood pressure response to locally applied cold to be a useful measure for estimating the degree of arteriosclerosis in both hypertensive and non-hypertensive patients.

Pathogenesis. Only a brief outline will be given here of the immense investigative effort which continues to go into the etiology of EH. In this search, two features of the disease have loomed prominently, *viz.,* the strong genetic susceptibility and the self-perpetuating nature of the disease.

The genetic susceptibility is clear not only from clinical records but from the emergence through inbreeding of spontaneously hypertensive rats (SHR) whose disease strongly resembles EH. In other genetic studies, rat strains have been developed which are supersensitive to salt feeding, *i.e.,* in whom hypertension will occur on salt diets which are innocuous to normal rats.

The concept of the almost inevitable progression of the disease is fostered by the experimental evidence that hypertension begets arteriosclerosis, which in turn begets further pressure elevation. But what starts the process is not known. Among the many explanations for the initiation of EH are the *neurogenic theory,* proposed by Folkow and others, the *arterial pressure-urinary output* theory of Guyton and the *regulatory imbalance* or mosaic theory of Page. Evidence is not yet at hand to warrant unequivocal acceptance of any single theory.

The *neurogenic theory* is supported in part by the considerable evidence that the nervous system is much involved in the regulation of arterial blood pressure. For example, hypertension can be produced by denervation of the arterial baroceptors, by chronic hypothalamic stimulation (Fig. 15-4) and by long-term psychogenic, emotional-frustration experiments in animals. Folkow believes that in susceptible individuals, there is a sensitivity of the arterial smooth muscle to continued sympathetic stimulation from the hypothalamic defense area, which in turn responds to continued psychogenic influence. This will gradually cause hypertrophy and an increased thickness of the media of these vessels, an increasing wall/lumen ratio, an inability of these vessels to dilate and an inevitable progressive increase in vascular resistance which leads to the hypertension.

From an extensive application of computer techniques to renal and arterial pressure control systems, Guyton has developed a theory for blood pressure control previously described in Chapter 10. This *arte-*

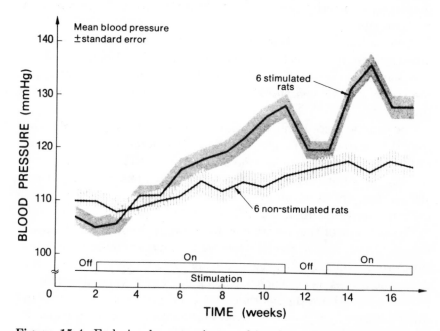

Figure 15-4. Enduring hypertension resulting from chronic stimulation of the hypothalamic defense area in the conscious rat. Stimulation was stopped during the 11th to 13th weeks. (From B. Folkow and E. H. Rubinstein, *Acta Physiol. Scand.* 68:48, 1966.)

rial pressure-urinary output theory proposes that the predominant long-term influence on the height of the arterial pressure is the urinary output of sodium and water, particularly the former. He suggests that even a minor disturbance in renal function can lead to a progressive elevation in arterial pressure because of the infinite gain of the system. Guyton's theory holds, therefore, that EH begins as a renovascular deficiency and continues because of the obligatory arterial pressure-urinary output relation.

Page's *regulatory imbalance theory* assumes that a steady state exists among a number of factors which regulate blood pressure (Fig. 15-5). The different factors contribute, in varying degrees, to the maintenance of balance. One or more of these variables may be changed in an independent manner to produce hypertension. The theory assumes that EH is a "multifactorial disease of regulation" and that no single underlying cause is to be expected since no one mechanism dominates the regulatory process.

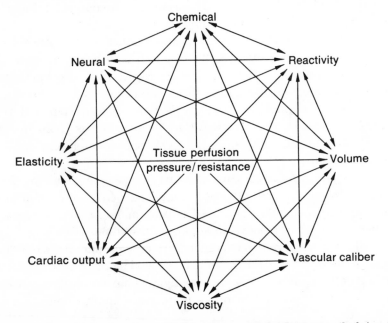

Figure 15-5. Mosaic octagon illustrating multiple factors underlying the pressure/resistance control of tissue perfusion. (From I. H. Page, *Circ. Res.* 34: 133, 1974. By permission of the American Heart Association, Inc.)

Treatment of Hypertension

Among cardiovascular disorders, there are few that require greater skill in differential diagnosis nor more diligent, constant attention to achieve successful treatment. Yet there are also very few in which the available treatment is as effective and the outlook as promising, provided the patient is cooperative. Because the symptoms are often minimal and the side effects of the drugs sometimes unpleasant, patients are frequently unwilling to follow their regimen.

The therapy for secondary types of hypertension is first of all directed at the specific cause. In the large exclusion group, *i.e.*, EH, general measures would be instituted such as reduction of internal and external stress (so far as possible) moderate restriction of calories, cholesterol, saturated fat and salt, and finally regular physical exercise within the limits of the patient's age and cardiovascular status. For specific therapy, it is sometimes possible to select antihypertensive medication with a mechanism of action that specifically fits the pressor mechanism involved. This usually means a combination of diuretics, sympathetic inhibitors and vasodilators.

Thiazide and Related Diuretics. These frequently form the basis of antihypertensive drug therapy. They are usually begun at moderate doses, the results followed, the dosage regulated and other agents added to achieve specific effects in individual patients. These drugs lower arterial pressure by blocking sodium reabsorption and thus causing salt and water depletion. Careful attention is given to side-effects which include potassium loss, elevated blood glucose and elevated uric acid.

Sympathetic Inhibitors. Guanethidine is a postganglionic blocking agent which prevents NE release; the main side-effect of guanethidine is postural hypotension. Also used is propranolol, a beta-adrenergic blocker which inhibits the renin-angiotensin system. "High renin" and "normal renin" hypertensives respond better to propranolol while "low renin" hypertensives (who have a lower incidence of heart attacks) respond better to diuretics; some investigators have recently advocated "renin-sodium profiling" in order to improve therapy selection for these patients.

Vasodilating Agents. Such agents as hydralazine or diazoxide, which relax vascular smooth muscle, are not used alone but mainly as adjuncts.

The mortality in hypertension, which results mainly from myocardial failure, stroke or renal failure, has in the last years been markedly reduced with the advent of effective antihypertensive drugs. Yet there is recent disconcerting evidence that while the lives of hypertensive patients are being prolonged, arteriosclerosis is still the cause of a high percentage of deaths; thus antihypertensive therapy is apparently blunting the disease but not preventing the eventual development of atherosclerosis. These findings are being further investigated.

CIRCULATORY SHOCK

General Characteristics and Classification

Circulatory shock is a failure of the circulation with decreased perfusion and/or inadequate oxygenation of the vital organs and cells of the body. It is due to trauma, blood loss, myocardial failure, infection or other serious bodily insult, and if untreated, has a tendency to progress toward general circulatory failure and death. Although the causes of circulatory shock are multiple, there are three main clinical types, *i.e., hypovolemic, cardiogenic* and *septic shock.*

In *hypovolemic shock,* a decrease in circulating blood volume is responsible for the fall in arterial pressure and in *cardiogenic shock* it is myocardial failure, *e.g.,* as a result of infarction, which causes the circulatory collapse. *Septic shock* often occurs incident to a massive infection, in which cardiac output and arterial pressure are usually normal or above normal, but the vital organs because of a metabolic defect are unable to extract adequate oxygen from the circulating blood.

While there are important clinical differences between the various types of shock, there are also many common features. A previously untreated patient after a severe trauma or blood loss will usually have a characteristic profound pallor of the skin and mucous membranes, there will be a cold sweat and a rapid, almost imperceptible, "thready" pulse (rate ≥ 140/min). The arterial pressure will be low (perhaps 85/60), the rectal temperature is often decreased to about 96 or 97° F. and respiration is feeble. The patient may be restless yet apathetic, and often semirational. Without early and proper treatment such a circulatory failure will frequently progress to irreversibility and death.

Among the earliest systematic investigations into the mechanism of circulatory shock were those of Dr. George W. Crile, a surgeon, who in

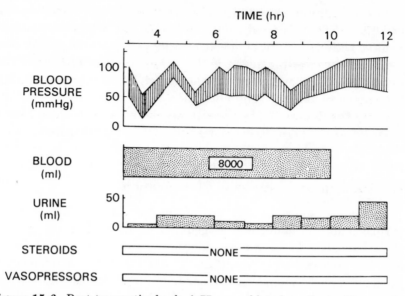

Figure 15-6. Post-traumatic shock. A 77-year-old male patient with a crushing injury of both legs and bilateral fractures of the femur, tibia and fibula; the patient, who had very little external blood loss, required blood infusions totalling 8000 ml over 7 hours. (From L. D. MacLean, J. H. Duff, and A. P. McLean, *Canad. Med. Assn. J.* 105:78, 1971.)

1899 reported his studies on shock in animals and the effect of different types of therapy. He described the low central venous pressure, the failure of venous return and cardiac output and the response to infusion. He believed the ultimate failure of the circulation to be due to sympathoadrenal exhaustion.

In 1918 Cannon and his colleagues studied shock in wounded soldiers in France; later in an extensive monograph they emphasized the correlation between low blood pressure and arterial acidosis as well as the beneficial effects of sodium bicarbonate infusion. These authors concluded that a histamine-like toxin, liberated from the traumatized cells, was the primary causative agent of the failure.

During the last 40 years, spurred particularly by the need for improved treatment of military casualties, extensive studies have been made of the pathogenesis and treatment of shock. As a result, shock therapy has improved dramatically; treatment is more "aggressive" with early and vigorous infusion of blood or blood substitutes and more reliable autonomic and inotropic agents are now available. Particularly effective has been the segregation of these patients into a special intensive care unit (ICU) or coronary care unit (CCU) with trained personnel and facilities for continuous on-line recording of vital cardiopulmonary parameters. As a consequence, the recovery rate in severe shock has been greatly improved.

In studies of severely shocked patients, it has been noted that in order to achieve hemodynamic stability, it is frequently necessary to infuse much greater amounts of fluid or blood than would be anticipated (Fig. 15-6). This is because of excessive fluid loss through hemorrhage, sequestration into certain capillary beds or diffusion into interstitial tissues.

Hypovolemic Shock

The pathophysiological changes and, therefore, the clinical picture, will vary somewhat in the different types of shock. In this section, hypovolemic shock, which is in a sense a prototype of clinical shock, will be described; later in the chapter some of the specific features of cardiogenic and septic shock will be discussed. Hypovolemic shock may result from hemorrhage, trauma, burns, excess radiation or any other injury which involves severe loss of body fluids, plasma or blood. In many of these conditions, *e.g.*, in burns or acute pancreatitis, the loss is not external but into the interstitial tissues; nonetheless it becomes unavailable to the cardiovascular system as circulating fluid.

Cardiovascular Changes. The circulatory alterations are due to the hypovolemia, and also, as will be noted later, to the compensatory changes resulting from the hypovolemia. The initial alterations are very similar to those seen early in hemorrhage, which were described in Chapter 13. In typical hypovolemic shock, the main circulatory effects are: (a) decrease in central and peripheral venous pressure, in circulating blood volume and in venous return; (b) decrease in cardiac output, with particular reduction in flow to the skin, splanchnic area and kidney; (c) decrease in arterial blood pressure (mean, systolic, diastolic and pulse pressure); (d) increased heart rate and myocardial contractility; (e) generalized vasoconstriction and venoconstriction with stagnant hypoxia; (f) hemodilution, with increased $Paco_2$ and decreased pH. Within a few hours there follows a leukocytosis, a nonspecific stress response whose mechanism is not known.

The typical progression of the circulatory changes can be illustrated in an experimental animal as shown in Figure 15-7. In this experiment, hypovolemic shock and hypotension were induced by hemorrhage; after a 2-hour interval, the blood was reinfused and additional periodic transfusion given. In spite of this the circulation failed progressively and the animal died. Whether the shock becomes irreversible is mainly dependent on the degree and duration of the hypotension; the possible cause of this irreversibility will be discussed later.

Compensatory Responses. The reactions to the stress—most of them reflex in nature—are an important part of the shock syndrome. The initial responses are directed particularly toward restoration of the two main deficiencies—the blood pressure and the blood volume.

Almost immediately, the decreased central venous volume (and pressure) will initiate autonomic cardiopulmonary reflexes, and the falling arterial and pulse pressure will induce strong arterial baroceptor responses (Chapter 10); these reflexes will result in tachycardia, increased myocardial contractility, widespread vasoconstriction and ve-

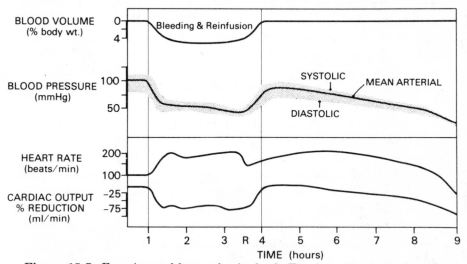

Figure 15-7. Experimental hemorrhagic shock. Two-hour hypovolemia and hypotension. Note the sharp fall in cardiac output (CO) and arterial pressure (AP), and rise in heart rate. With reinfusion of the withdrawn blood (at R), CO and AP recovered but later declined in spite of subsequent transfusion. (From C. J. Wiggers, *Physiology of Shock.* Cambridge, Mass.: Harvard University Press, 1950. Reprinted by permission.)

noconstriction, release of adrenal medullary catecholamines and hyperventilation. When acidosis becomes evident, the arterial chemoceptors will also be activated and add an additional pressor effect; in deep shock the CNS ischemic reflex will provoke a still more intense sympathetic vasoconstricton (Chapter 10).

These reflex responses will tend to restore both cardiac output and arterial pressure but they will not be maintained equally. As increasing fractions of blood volume are removed, the cardiac output will tend to fall, while arterial pressure may be temporarily maintained if the bleeding is not too rapid (Fig. 15-8).

Several important points should be noted from the graph in Figure 15-8. First, the maintenance of pressure at the expense of flow is the classic definition of resistance and the ratio of the two is a measure of the extent to which total vascular resistance is being mobilized, as was discussed in Chapter 2. However, while the mean arterial pressure is being maintained, the pulse pressure steadily declines; if the heart rate is not changing greatly, this would suggest (if cardiac output determinations are not available) that stroke volume and cardiac output are

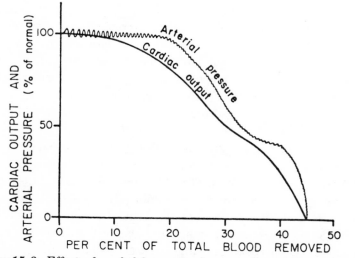

Figure 15-8. Effect of graded hemorrhage on cardiac output and arterial pressure. Early in the bleeding, cardiac output (CO) falls but arterial pressure (AP) is maintained. After withdrawal of about 20% of the blood volume both AP and CO decline rapidly. (From A. C. Guyton, *Textbook of Medical Physiology,* 5th ed. Philadelphia: W. B. Saunders Co., 1976.)

declining. Finally, the graph indicates that with about 15% of the blood volume removed, the bleeding still continuing and the cardiac output declining, the mean arterial pressure may still be relatively normal; thus in such a situation, the mean arterial pressure is not a good index of the state of the circulation. For this reason, pulse pressure, heart rate, central venous pressure, urine output and other clinical signs must also be carefully monitored during shock.

Systemic vascular resistance is approximately doubled and pulmonary vascular resistance is increased about 5-fold in severe shock. As mentioned earlier, the sympathetic vasconstriction is selective; constriction of the skin is responsible for the pallor and the renal vasoconstriction reduces glomerular filtration pressure, resulting in oliguria (decreased urine flow) or, if severe, anuria (cessation of urine output). The vasoconstriction in skeletal muscle and in the splanchnic area and the widespread venoconstriction will mobilize blood from these "reservoirs"; this mobilization and the simultaneous shrinking of the general vascular capacity are very important aids to venous return and cardiac output.

Within minutes after hemorrhage or trauma, there is also a prompt tendency to restore *vascular volume,* mainly through: (a) influx of interstitial fluid into the capillaries through reduction of intracapillary hydrostatic pressure (Chapter 8); (b) renal vasoconstriction which aside from reducing glomerular filtration pressure and urine output, will also activate the renin-angiotensin-aldosterone mechanism (Chapters 13 and 15, Renal Circulation) and thus increase sodium and, therefore also water reabsorption from the renal tubules; and (c) reduced atrial pressure and activation of osmoreceptors will stimulate the hypothalamus and prompt the release of vasopressin (ADH) from the posterior pituitary gland (Chapter 15, Renal Circulation); the latter will increase the reabsorption of water from the renal tubules. Some compensatory responses are shown graphically in Figure 15-9.

Metabolic and Endocrine Changes. While the cardiovascular fluctuations in shock are dramatic and because of their urgency receive more attention, the metabolic and endocrine changes are in the long run, equally if not more significant since it is likely that irreversibility is due primarily to metabolic failure. The primary metabolic changes in moderate or severe hypovolemic shock are:

1. Decreased metabolic rate and body temperature.

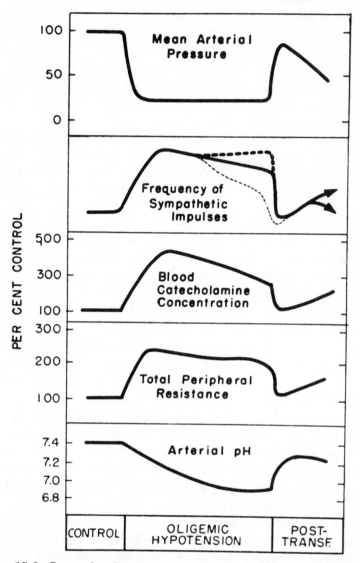

Figure 15-9. Sympathoadrenal and blood pH responses to experimental hemorrhagic shock. The experimental procedure was similar to that shown in Figure 15-7 with reinfusion of the blood after the hypotensive period. In late shock, the frequency of sympathetic impulses may take different time courses as shown. Note the gradual decline in impulse frequency, catecholamine concentration and vascular resistance and the progressive development of acidosis. (From S. Chien, *Physiol. Rev.* 47:252, 1967.)

2. Alteration in carbohydrate metabolism: (a) an initial hypergly-cemia, due to release of epinephrine; later in shock, hypoglycemia may occur because of depletion of hepatic glycogen and failure of gluconeo-genesis; (b) anaerobic glycolysis with increase in blood lactate and pyruvate. There is also depletion of high energy phosphates, especially in the liver and kidney; however, those of brain and heart are well maintained.

3. Protein catabolism: (a) increase in blood amino acid nitrogen indicating increased protein catabolism due to the stagnant hypoxia; (b) decrease in blood urea associated with a decline in deamination function of the liver due to hepatic ischemia; (c) increase in liver and blood ammonia.

4. Blood: increase in $Paco_2$ and decrease in pH, but the Pao_2 is usually well maintained; hemodilution, except in burns and in some cases of severe trauma, in which the hematocrit is high; increase in plasma catecholamines, 17 hydroxyketosteroids and blood K^+.

The metabolic changes are mainly the result of (a) a generalized stagnant hypoxia, during which the intracellular Po_2 becomes very low with a resultant peripheral anaerobiosis, and (b) increased neuroen-docrine activity, particularly of the sympathoadrenal and anterior pituitary-adrenal cortical systems.

Cardiogenic Shock

Cardiogenic shock usually denotes insufficient output of the heart despite an adequate ventricular filling pressure. While such a situation results primarily from myocardial infarction (MI), this type of shock can and does occur from a mechanical cardiac defect such as pericardial effusion (tamponade), a sudden valve failure or as a later development in septic or hypovolemic shock.

In the classical case, however, it will result from an MI. Significant arterial hypotension and shock will develop if the myocardial damage is sufficient (about 30 to 40% of the myocardial mass) and if the systemic vascular resistance is not adequate to maintain the arterial pressure. The net result will depend mainly on (a) the effect of the MI on myocardial pump function, and (b) the reflex response to the myocardial injury.

The reflex sympathetic vasoconstrictor response is of paramount importance for survival. As mentioned in Chapter 14, the vascular reflex reaction to MI is not generally predictable, with pressor and depressor responses occurring with about equal frequency. The basic mechanisms involved are not clear but it appears that cardiocardiac reflexes are very importantly concerned in the process.

Cardiac vagal receptors reportedly induce both pressor and depressor responses; on the other hand, recent studies have shown that afferent impulses from coronary vessels and from mechanoreceptors in the ischemic canine and primate ventricle also travel in the dorsal sympathetic chain. These fibers can carry pain sensation but even more important, they can apparently inhibit sympathetic vasoconstrictors.

Obviously the vasomotor and cardiac centers of the medulla are subjected to conflicting influences; aside from the afferent cardiac impulses which are variable (but apparently mainly depressor), the remaining cardiopulmonary afferents and the arterial baroceptors are strongly pressor. The net response is the result of the integration of these (and other) impulses by the medullary centers. An interesting recent finding is that efferent constrictor impulses to upper and lower limb skeletal muscle may elicit different responses, raising the possibility of more specific efferent control of vascular resistance than has been ordinarily visualized.

The pumping efficiency of the ventricle will be considerably influenced by the degree of myocardial damage as well as its effect on ventricular compliance; the relationship of the compliance change to fluid therapy will be discussed later. With a compromised myocardium, the reflex vasoconstriction is usually the main determinant of arterial pressure; the arterial pressure in turn is critical, not only from the standpoint of the shock state, but because of the possible damaging effect of continued hypotension on enlargement of the infarct area.

Septic Shock

Septic shock is usually the result of a severe infection and bacteremia, often with Gram-negative organisms. The patient frequently has an increased central venous pressure (CVP) and cardiac output, hyperventilation and alkalosis along with hypotension, tachycardia and a low peripheral vascular resistance.

In contrast to this hyperdynamic state, there is also a form of hypodynamic septic shock in which there is a decreased CVP and cardiac output, increased peripheral resistance and cold, cyanotic extremities.

There is in septic shock a lactacidemia with a low arterial-mixed venous oxygen gradient indicating inadequate delivery of oxygen to the tissues. The cause of this deficiency is not certain but apparently involves a basic metabolic defect, perhaps due to a circulating toxin which interferes with cellular oxygen utilization. While septic shock is frequently the direct result of infection, it may also occur as an aftermath of cardiogenic or hypovolemic shock, perhaps because of temporary deleterious effect of the latter on the body's bacterial defense mechanisms. Unlike the preceding forms of shock, septic shock is often associated with other pathological complications such as acute respiratory failure with pulmonary edema and disseminated intravascular coagulation (DIC); the latter is an extensive disorder of the blood clotting mechanism characterized by frequent occurrence of microemboli.

Pathogenesis of Circulatory Shock

The hemodynamic and metabolic changes in early hypovolemic and cardiogenic shock are the result of the low cardiac output, hypotension and generalized stagnant hypoxia. However, in many cases of septic shock the cardiac output is normal or even elevated but the cellular damage leads to similar metabolic results.

The search for the mechanism of the later changes in shock, particularly the irreversibility, has been unsuccessful in spite of enormous research efforts. Two special difficulties complicate the shock problem; first, as Wiggers has pointed out, shock not only stops the machine, but wrecks the machinery; so many processes are simultaneously affected that it is difficult to determine which is the primary disorder. The result has been innumerable theories concerning the irreversibility with the evidence frequently being only circumstantial. The second difficulty lies in finding a common denominator for a process which can be initiated in many different ways and in which the only endpoint is a fatality. However, while a single cause has not yet been found, our understanding of circulatory shock has been considerably advanced in recent years.

Site of the Failure in Shock. From the standpoint of etiology, many studies have been concerned with the question of which organ or system initiates the irreversibility; other investigators have concentrated on which process might be responsible. In earlier studies, the excessive splanchnic vasoconstriction and hepatic ischemia, especially in experimental animals, drew attention to the liver as a possible critical site. The role of other organs has also been carefully studied. Selkurt has published an excellent review of the role of the kidney in shock and Lefer and Spath, after extensive investigations, have suggested the importance of pancreatic ischemia in the genesis of shock.

The main issue of the failure site has, however, revolved around the question of whether it is basically of cardiac or peripheral circulatory origin. Jones *et al.* have advocated the primary role of the heart; Zweifach and Froneck, in their extensive analysis of shock mechanisms, stated that in their opinion, the issue was unsettled but favored the view that peripheral failure was responsible.

There is considerable evidence to indicate the critical importance of venous return and particularly of the neural control of the circulation for shock survival. Stekiel and his colleagues recently have reported adrenergic neurotransmitter depletion in mesenteric arteries in hemorrhagic shock and believe that loss of such compensatory vasoconstriction may be a key defect. Kovach and his group have found marked reduction of blood flow and loss of responsiveness in the hypothalamus and reticular formation of dogs in hypovolemic shock and have indicated the potential importance of this central neurogenic influence on irreversibility.

Metabolic and Biological Processes in Shock. Some investigators have focused their efforts, not on a target organ but on a basic metabolic process, in order to study its role in shock development. While a number of metabolic deficiencies have been identified, none of these have thus far been proved to be an instigating factor in the irreversibility. Studies by Filkins and co-workers and Hinshaw and others have emphasized the importance of certain aspects of carbohydrate metabolism, particularly in endotoxin shock.

Irreversibility is usually characterized by a marked hypoglycemia and a profound depression of gluconeogenesis; shock mortality is also found to be increased in situations of enhanced insulin secretion, suggesting an important role for hyperinsulinemia as well as hypoglycemia in endotoxin and perhaps septic shock.

The Reticuloendothelial System (RES) in Shock. In early studies, Zweifach and others noted a correlation between RES function and the mortality from trauma, as well as increased shock mortality following RES blockade. Filkins *et al.* demonstrated that administration of zymosan, a yeast extract with potent RES-modulating properties, significantly lowered the mortality of rats to traumatic shock. Loegering and Saba have reported that in experimental shock, there was a depression of RES phagocytic function; the evidence indicates that both humoral and cellular factors may be involved in the decreased functional capacity of the RES in shock. It has been suggested that such a decline in the body defense mechanism may play a role in septic shock and particularly in its occurrence as a sequela to other types of circulatory failure.

Toxic Factors in Shock. A number of circulating toxins have been proposed as causative agents for the irreversibility in shock. Fine and his colleagues were the first to suggest that bacterial endotoxins, absorbed from the ischemic gut might play a role in the pathophysiology of shock. This view was given support by the finding that very small doses of endotoxin could produce in experimental animals a circulatory failure resembling hypovolemic and traumatic shock. While the overall role of endotoxins in shock is uncertain, some investigators believe they are concerned in the circulatory failure in bacteremia, particularly of the Gram-negative type.

Lefer and co-workers have accumulated considerable evidence for a causal relationship between a myocardial depressant factor (MDF) and mortality in experimental shock. MDF is a low molecular weight, dialyzable polypeptide apparently produced in the pancreas and recoverable from the blood of animals suffering shock. As a result of a large number of systematic studies, these investigators have shown that MDF has not only a strong myocardial depressant effect but has splanchnic vasoconstrictor and other actions as well. However, the role of MDF in human shock is still unknown.

Lysosomes in Shock. Following the pioneer work of De Duve on the role of lysosomes in cellular function, investigations have been made of their possible role in shock. Studies have indicated that hypoxia and mechanical trauma cause disruption of lysosomes *in vitro*; furthermore after hemorrhage, endotoxin injection or trauma, lysosomal proteases escape from ischemic cells and are found in high concentration in the plasma. Some investigators have ascribed the role of the RES in shock to the fact that RES tissue is rich in lysosomes. The interaction of proteases from disrupted lysosomes with plasma proteins is thought to be the source of several protein derivatives such as MDF which are known to have vasoactive properties. Although the evidence is controversial, some investigators have proposed that lysosomes may play a basic role in the etiology of lethal shock as outlined in Figure 15-10.

As is evident from the preceding, the important question of the cause of irreversibility is as yet unanswered, at least in human shock.

Treatment of Shock

Fluid Replacement and Central Venous Pressure. Because in the great majority of shock patients, there is a fluid deficit, treatment is first of all directed toward replacement therapy with plasma, blood substitutes or whole blood depending on individual needs. The monitoring of such therapy is often done *via* central venous pressure (CVP). Clinical CVP monitoring usually refers to central vena caval or right atrial pressure and therefore is a general index of *right* ventricular filling pressure and *right* ventricular end-diastolic pressure (VEDP).

As discussed in Chapter 2, pressure in the central veins (as in any blood vessel) depends on the distensibility (or compliance) of the vessel and the volume contained. Heightened sympathetic tone will decrease the distensibility; however, at any given distensibility level, CVP will be dependent on the contained volume which will, in turn,

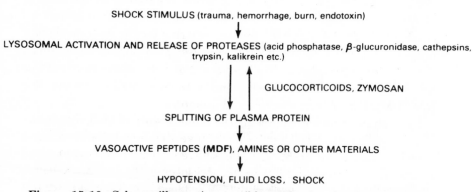

Figure 15-10. Schema illustrating possible mechanism for the development of irreversible shock. Glucocorticoids and zymosan (an extract of brewers' yeast) have both been shown to lower mortality in experimental shock, presumably through their ability to stabilize lysosomal membranes.

reflect the balance of inflow and outflow. If there is no abnormality of right ventricular function nor of intrathoracic pressure, CVP will be an index of venous return and serve as a rough guide to circulating blood volume and the need for fluid replacement therapy. CVP is normally about 5 to 10 cm saline and in shock usually is below 3 to 4 cm saline. The goal is to achieve about 8 to 10 cm saline CVP with additional fluid, provided other signs do not contraindicate such treatment. The general objective is to improve ventricular function through greater diastolic filling (the Starling effect).

Monitoring of Ventricular Function in Cardiogenic Shock. In cardiogenic shock, in contrast to the above, factors other than circulating blood volume will influence ventricular filling pressure and, therefore, must be taken into consideration. As mentioned in Chapter 14, after an MI with left ventricular involvement, there will be a gradual decrease in LV compliance with a concomitant rise in LVEDP. The latter development is generally beneficial since it improves ventricular function, but it has two potential disadvantages. Since the ventricular diastolic curve rises steeply (Fig. 14-4), diastolic volume and, therefore, stroke volume will be limited. The second additional factor is that a rising LVEDP increases the possibility of pulmonary congestion.

In such a situation, left ventricular monitoring obviously becomes of prime importance in the treatment of cardiogenic shock. However, CVP is a poor reflection of LVEDP. Fortunately, Swan, Ganz and their colleagues reported in 1970 the development of a double-lumen, flow-directed catheter which could be guided *via* an external vein, into the pulmonary artery without fluoroscopy. This permits the monitoring of pulmonary arterial pressure for the detection of any developing pulmonary congestion and by "wedging" of the catheter into a pulmonary arterial branch, also provides a reasonable estimate of left atrial pressure and thus of left ventricular filling pressure.

Using this technique, clinical studies have indicated that fluid replacement therapy can safely be continued up to left ventricular filling pressures of about 20 to 24 mm Hg. This will provide a reasonable level for improvement of ventricular function *via* the Starling effect without undue risk of inducing pulmonary congestion. Thus in cardiogenic shock, a pulmonary artery catheter as well as a central venous catheter is usually employed. In this way both right and left sides of the heart may be monitored.

Intraaortic Balloon Counterpulsation (IABC). In very severe shock in which arterial pressure cannot be maintained despite all available methods, additional circulatory support is sometimes given by introduction *via* catheter of an inflatable balloon into the upper thoracic aorta. The balloon is inflated during diastole and rapidly deflated at the end of diastole. Thus diastolic pressure is increased which assists coronary flow, and systolic peak pressure is decreased which reduces the afterload work of the left ventricle. With this procedure, cardiac output is increased with relatively little change in mean arterial pressure. Counterpulsation has proven helpful in certain circumstances in achieving hemodynamic stability (Fig. 15-11).

Specific Therapy. A number of vasoactive substances have come into increasing use in shock. Adrenergic agents, particularly those with beta mimetic effect such as isoproterenol, are used as adjunctive

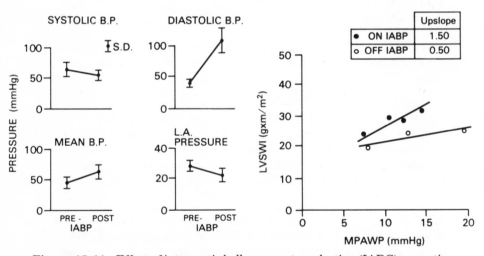

Figure 15-11. Effect of intraaortic balloon counterpulsation (IABC) on aortic and left atrial pressure and left ventricular stroke work index. *Left,* values immediately before and after IABC; *Right,* the relationship of mean pulmonary artery wedge pressure (MPAWP) and left ventricular stroke work index (LVSWI) before and after IABC. In a critically ill patient, MPAWP is equivalent to left atrial filling pressure. Note the improved ventricular function during IABC. (From R. L. Berger, V. K. Saini, T. J. Ryan, D. M. Sokol, and J. F. Keefe, *J. Thor. Cardiovasc. Surg.* 66:906, 1973; and R. D. Weisel, R. L. Berger, and H. B. Hechtman, *N. Engl. J. Med.* 292:682, 1975. Reprinted by permission from the New England Journal of Medicine.)

therapy to improve cardiac contractility. Dopamine, a naturally occurring catecholamine precursor, has been found useful, particularly in septic shock. Dopamine has both beta- and alpha-adrenergic action; aside from the cardiac effect, the beta action will induce mesenteric and renal vasodilation, the latter sometimes being effective in increasing urine flow. The alpha action produces mild vasoconstriction.

Digitalis is sometimes used to improve cardiac contractility. Although the exact action of glucocorticoids in shock is not known, they are occasionally effective in some cases of otherwise intractable shock.

It should be emphasized that the treatment of shock is highly complex. The few general principles described above are intended only to illustrate some of the pathophysiology involved and not to serve as a guide to therapy.

REFERENCES

Hypertension

ANTONACCIO, M. S. (Ed.): *Cardiovascular Pharmacology.* New York: Raven Press, 1977.

BROD, J., V. FENCL, Z. HEJL, AND J. JIRKA: Circulatory changes underlying blood pressure elevation during acute emotional stress. *Clin. Sci.* 18:269, 1959.

CHARVAT, J., P. L. DELL, P. FOLKOW, AND B. FOLKOW: Mental factors and cardiovascular diseases. *Cardiologia* 44:124–141, 1964.

CHOBANIAN, A. V.: Pathophysiology of systemic hypertension. In *Clinical Cardiovascular Physiology,* ed. by H. J. Levine. New York: Grune & Stratton Inc., 1976.

COLEMAN, T. G., A. W. COWLEY, JR., AND A. C. GUYTON: Experimental hypertension and the long-term control of arterial pressure. In *Cardiovascular Physiology,* Vol. 1, MTP International Review of Science, ed. by A. C. Guyton and C. E. Jones. Baltimore: University Park Press, 1974.

DEJONG, W., AND A. P. PROVOST (Eds.): *Hypertension and Brain Mechanisms.* Amsterdam: Elsevier/North Holland Biomedical Press, 1977.

FINK, G. D., AND M. J. BRODY: Neurogenic control of renal circulation in hypertension. *Fed. Proc.* 37:1202–1208, 1978.

FROLICH, E. D.: Cardiovascular pathophysiology of essential hypertension. In *The Peripheral Circulations,* ed. by R. Zelis. New York: Grune & Stratton Inc., 1975.

FROLICH, E. D., R. C. TARAZI, M. ULRYCH, H. P. DUNSTAN, AND I. H. PAGE: Tilt test for investigating a neural component in hypertension. *Circulation* 36:387–393, 1967.

GAUER, O. H., AND J. P. HENRY: Circulatory basis of fluid volume control. *Physiol. Rev.* 43:423–481, 1963.

HULL, D. H., R. A. WOLTHUIS, T. CORTESE, M. R. LONGO, AND J. H. TRIEBWASSER: Borderline hypertension versus normotension and differential response to orthostatic stress. *Am. Heart J.* 94:414–420, 1977.

ITSKOVITZ, H. D., M. S. KOCHAR, A. J. ANDERSON, AND A. A. RIMM: Patterns of blood pressure in Milwaukee. *J.A.M.A.* 238:864–868, 1977.

LARAGH, J. H. (Ed.) Symposium on hypertension: mechanisms and management. *Am. J. Med.* 52:565–578, 1972 (#5).

LARAGH, J. H., R. L. LETCHER, AND T. G. PICKERING. Renin profiling for diagnosis and treatment of hypertension. *J.A.M.A.* 241:151–156, 1979.

MANCIA, G., J. LUDBROOK, A. FERRARI, L. GREGORINI, AND A. ZANCHETTI: Baroceptor reflexes in human hypertension. *Circ. Res.* 43:170–177, 1978.

MCGIFF, J. C., K. CROWSHAW, AND H. D. ITSKOVITZ: Prostaglandins and renal function. *Fed. Proc.* 33:39–47, 1974.

PAGE, I. H.: Arterial hypertension in retrospect. *Circ. Res.* 34:133–142, 1974.

PICKERING, SIR GEORGE: Hypertension—definitions, natural histories and consequences. *Am. J. Cardiol.* 52:570–583, 1972.

SAFAR, M. E., Y. A. WEISS, J. A. LEVENSON, G. M. LONDON, AND P. L. MILLIEZ: Hemodynamic study of eighty-five patients with borderline hypertension. *Am. J. Cardiol.* 31:315–319, 1973.

VOUDOUKIS, I. J.: Exaggerated cold pressor responses in patients with atherosclerotic vascular disease. *Angiology* 22:57–62, 1971.

Circulatory Shock

BECKMAN, C. B., A. S. GEHA, G. L. HAMMOND, AND A. E. BAVE: Results and complications of intra-aortic balloon counter-pulsaton. *Ann. Thorac. Surg.* 24:550–559, 1977.

BUCHANAN, B. J., AND J. P. FILKINS: Hypoglycemic depression of RES function. *Am. J. Physiol.* 231:265–269, 1976.

FILKINS, J. P., J. M. LUBITZ, AND J. J. SMITH: The effect of zymosan and glucan on the reticuloendothelial system and on resistance to traumatic shock. *Angiology* 15:465–470, 1964.

FILKINS, J. P., B. J. BUCHANAN, AND R. P. CORNELL: Hepatic carbohydrate metabolic alterations during endotoxic and traumatic shock. *Circ. Shock* 2:129–135, 1975.

FILNER, B., J. S. KARLINER, AND P. O. DAILY: Favorable influence of dopamine on left ventricular performance in patients refractory to discontinuation of cardiopulmonary bypass. *Circ. Shock* 4:223–230, 1977.

FINE, J., S. RUTENBURG, AND F. B. SCHWEINBURG: The role of the RES in hemorrhagic shock. *J. Exp. Med.* 110:547–569, 1959.

GUNNAR, R. M., H. S. LOEB, AND S. A. JOHNSON: Cardiogenic shock. In *Clinical Cardiovascular Physiology,* ed. by H. J. Levine. New York: Grune & Stratton Inc., 1976.

HINSHAW, L. B.: Concise review: The role of glucose in endotoxin shock. *Circ. Shock* 3:6–10, 1976.

JONES, C. E., E. E. SMITH, AND J. W. CROWELL: Cardiac output and physiological mechanisms in circulatory shock. In *Cardiovascular Physiology,* MTP International Review of Science, ed. by A. C. Guyton and C. E. Jones Baltimore: University Park Press, 1974.

KOSTREVA, D. R., G. L. HESS, E. J. ZUPERKU, J. NEUMARK, R. L. COON, AND J. P. KAMPINE: Cardiac responses to stimulation of thoracic afferents in the primate and canine. *Am. J. Physiol.* 231:1279–1284, 1976.

KOVACH, A. G. B., AND P. SANDOR: Cerebral blood flow and brain function during hypotension and shock. *Physiol Rev.* 38:571–596, 1976.

LEFER, A. M., AND J. A. SPATH: Pharmacologic basis for the treatment of circulatory shock. In *Cardiovascular Pharmacology,* ed. by M. Antonaccio. New York: Raven Press, 1977.

LOEGERING, D. J., AND T. M. SABA: Hepatic Kupffer cell dysfunction during hemorrhagic shock. *Circ. Res.* 3:107–113, 1976.

LOMBARD, J. H., D. J. LOEGERING, AND W. J. STEKIEL: Effects of prolonged hemorrhagic hypotensive stress on catecholamine concentration of mesenteric blood vessels. *Blood Vessels* 14:212–228, 1977.

McLEAN, L. D.: Shock: Causes and management of circulatory collapse. In *Textbook of Surgery,* 11th ed., ed. by D. C. Sabiston, Philadelphia: 1977.

NELSON, A. W., AND H. SWAN: Hemorrhage: Responses determining survival. *Circ. Shock* 1:273–285, 1974.

SELKURT, E. E. Current status of renal circulation in experimental shock. *Circ. Shock* 1:3–15, 1974.

SMITH, J. J., D. J. LOEGERING, D. J. McDERMOTT, AND M. L. BONIN: The role of lysosomal hydrolases in the mechanism of shock. In *Neurohumoral and Metabolic Aspects of Injury,* ed. by A. G. B. Kovach, H. B. Stoner, and J. J. Spitzer. New York: Plenum Publishing Co., 1973.

SWAN, H. J., W. GANZ, J. FORRESTER, H. MARCUS, G. DIAMOND, AND D. CHONETTE: Catheterization of the heart in man with use of a flow-directed balloon-tipped catheter. *N. Engl. J. Med.* 283:447–450, 1970.

ZWEIFACH, B., AND A. FRONECK: Interplay of central and peripheral factors in irreversible hemorrhagic shock. *Prog. Cardiovasc. Dis.* 18:147–180, 1975.

INDEX

Pages numbered in **boldface** indicate more definitive discussion of the topics.

Pages numbered in **boldface** indicate more definitive discussion of the topics.

Pages numbered in **boldface** indicate more definitive discussion of the topics.

Pages numbered in **boldface** indicate more definitive discussion of the topics.

Pages numbered in **boldface** indicate more definitive discussion of the topics.

Pages numbered in **boldface** indicate more definitive discussion of the topics.

Pages numbered in **boldface** indicate more definitive discussion of the topics.

Pages numbered in **boldface** indicate more definitive discussion of the topics.

Pages numbered in **boldface** indicate more definitive discussion of the topics.

Pages numbered in **boldface** indicate more definitive discussion of the topics.

Pages numbered in **boldface** indicate more definitive discussion of the topics.

Pages numbered in **boldface** indicate more definitive discussion of the topics.

Pages numbered in **boldface** indicate more definitive discussion of the topics.

Pages numbered in **boldface** indicate more definitive discussion of the topics.

Pages numbered in **boldface** indicate more definitive discussion of the topics.

Pages numbered in **boldface** indicate more definitive discussion of the topics.